Doctors Choice

Doctor's CHOICE

A Hard-Working Doctor's Guide to Creating a Life of Freedom

Maritta Philp, MD

NEW YORK

LONDON • NASHVILLE • MELBOURNE • VANCOUVER

Doctors Choice

A Hard Working Doctor's Guide to Creating a Life of Freedom

Published in New York, New York, by Morgan James Publishing in partnership with Difference Press. Morgan James is a trademark of Morgan James, LLC. www.MorganJamesPublishing.com

The Morgan James Speakers Group can bring authors to your live event. For more information or to book an event visit The Morgan James Speakers Group at www.TheMorganJamesSpeakersGroup.com.

ISBN 9781683508199 paperback
ISBN 9781683508205 eBook
Library of Congress Control Number: 2017916532

Cover Design by:
Rachel Lopez
www.r2cdesign.com

Interior Design by:
Chris Treccani
www.3dogcreative.net

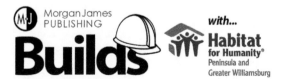

In an effort to support local communities, raise awareness and funds, Morgan James Publishing donates a percentage of all book sales for the life of each book to Habitat for Humanity Peninsula and Greater Williamsburg.

Get involved today! Visit
www.MorganJamesBuilds.com

Dedication

*To my mother,
who stood by me and loved me
through thick and thin.*

Table of Contents

Foreword

I first met Maritta when she came to train with me in one of my Rapid Transformational Therapy courses, and I was delighted when she asked me to write the foreword for her first book.

What makes Maritta extraordinary is the breadth of her knowledge and skills. Not only is she a medical doctor, she is also a skilled Rapid Transformational Therapist and psychotherapist with a real passion to make a profound difference to her clients, empowering them to step into an extraordinary life.

Her honesty about her experience working as a doctor is refreshing and at times shocking, as she tells of the pressure and stress that she and many of her colleagues have been and continue to be exposed to.

Her book is written for doctors who feel overwhelmed by the pressures they are facing every day, not knowing whether to stay or to go; to change how they work or to simply continue as they are while paying a high price.

In truth, this book would be useful for anyone feeling stuck and overwhelmed in their career or life in general, as the tools Maritta is teaching are universal and easily implemented.

The core of this book is a step-by-step guide to identify what you really want, what your values are, and how you can manifest your vision.

Her book is easy to read and filled with simple yet powerful exercises. Maritta's knowledge of the science behind many of our habits and behaviors is sound and helpful in understanding why we can get stuck and may find change difficult. She offers tools that make that change easy and manageable, without feeling overwhelmed.

Brimming with easy to use strategies, this book contains the knowledge that a reader needs to make a real change in their life and overcome whatever it is that keeps them stuck.

As a successful therapist and author myself, I have been aware of the importance of the material in Maritta's book for many years. I teach this material along with hypnotherapy and other skills to therapists around the world, who have phenomenal success with their clients, often changing lives in a single session.

The concepts that Maritta shares in *Doctor's Choice* are very powerful, as they can empower anyone to lead an extraordinary life. Read with an open heart, and prepare to take the first steps toward your new, fulfilling life.

Marisa Peer
www.marisapeer.com
www.rapidtransformationaltherapy.com
Author of:

Ultimate Confidence
You Can Be Thin
Trying to Get Pregnant (and Succeeding)
You Can Be Younger

The Typical Story

I know your story. It is my story, too.

I will tell you more about my story in a little while. It might be different in some of the details, but overall there will be more similarities than differences. We are all in the same boat. We all have similar experiences. We all face similar pressures.

You are a doctor and you are struggling with your work and your life. You picked up this book because you are considering quitting your practice. Perhaps this is the right decision, but it might not be. But you know for sure that the pressure is too much and that something must change.

Perhaps this change simply means identifying a healthier way to work. This could mean fewer hours, less pressure, a different post. Or it could mean a complete change of career and leaving medicine behind. These are big decisions, and there is a lot at stake: your life, your happiness, your future.

You work very hard. You have trained for decades to get to where you are right now. You started out loving your job and your patients, and helping them was the main driver for you, giving you satisfaction and meaning. It was so much more than a job: It was a calling, a vocation.

But over time this has been changing. You are feeling more and more worn out, tired, and exhausted. You're rushing through a caseload that continuously increases in both volume and complexity. You find that you cannot provide the quality of care you really want to; there simply is not enough time in the day; there is not enough of you.

You also find that your patients demand so much more of you now, but the system is not designed to cope with that demand. The system is based on need, not want.

You expend so much energy at work that there is little left for yourself, your loved ones, and the things you love to do. The joy and passion you once felt are slowly trickling out of your life, and you are now content to survive until the next weekend. You would love to be able to spend more quality time with your children and partner, cook homemade meals, look after your health, exercise more, but all you can muster is the energy to order takeout and watch TV.

That was my life, until I decided that I no longer wanted to experience that kind of daily pressure and drudgery.

Pressure

This kind of pressure has a price and we all pay it. We may pay in different currencies, though.

I had a colleague, for instance, who seemed to cope very well, until it emerged that he took prescription drugs and used alcohol to deal with the stress. His position at work became untenable and he had to leave. This increased the pressure on his colleagues significantly, and the practice is now struggling to manage. Another colleague collapsed at his desk at work and could not be resuscitated. He only had a few years before his planned retirement. He had a wife and young child. Yet another colleague retired, having felt ill and suffered with headaches for some years. It emerged he had a very rare form of brain tumor, and he died within two years of retirement.

We all know stories like these. Sadly, they are quite commonplace.

I came to realize that living life in this fashion is very unhealthy, and the price will be paid sooner or later. You cannot keep giving and never receiving. Just like you cannot keep breathing out and never take a breath in.

There are many reasons why we do what we do, why we have chosen a career that centers around caring for others. These are likely the same reasons why so often we feel stuck and unable to break free. We will explore these reasons in much more detail later in the book.

Identity

Some of these reasons have to do with our identities as doctors. This identity can be all-encompassing, especially since we have invested so much time, energy, passion, love, sweat, and tears into becoming doctors. Years of study and exams, nights and weekends on call, sacrificing time with our friends and loved ones, all to pursue this goal. Something we have fought for so hard is not given up easily.

Most doctors are so caught up in the hamster wheel of daily work that there is no time to reflect and consider the options we have. We feel obligated and pressured, and often there are feelings of guilt and shame around doing something we *want* to do, rather than something required of us. Somehow it seems a selfish thing to do. Or we simply feel there is nothing else we can do; no other career choice makes sense. Are we not getting a bit old to make such a change? Some of us might feel trapped in a golden cage, and financial worry keeps us locked in there.

There are so many reasons to leave things as they are. If only the price was not quite so high.

Something Needs to Change

The truth is that something needs to change. We simply cannot continue on the road of overwork we are on. Where will it lead? Will it really help our patients in the longer term? I don't think so. As a patient, I would much prefer to see a doctor who is well-rested and healthy, and who enjoys spending time in the consultation with me. I don't believe that a doctor who is overwhelmed, anxious, depressed, or stressed out can provide the same quality of care as a doctor who enjoys life, is healthy, and full of energy and enthusiasm for her job and her patient.

Of course, the situation is complex and there are other drivers. We live in an age of austerity. The government agenda and lack of funding in the health care system have a massive influence over the conditions in which we work.

Ultimately, none of this needs to make a difference in your choices. This book is not about departmental spending, government policy, or political agendas. This book is about you. Only you and what is important to you.

This Is All About You

I want you to know that there is a different way.

There are steps you can take to take back power and control. Steps which allow you to identify what it is that you really want, to find joy and passion again in your life. It will mean, though, that something must change. You cannot expect to keep doing the same thing over and over again and suddenly stumble upon a different outcome. A different outcome requires different thoughts, beliefs, emotions, and actions.

Only you can decide what these changes will look like. The steps in this book will help you identify the cost you will be paying should you decide to carry on as you are. It will teach you the tools you need to discover what it is that you really want, and enable you to take the next steps on that journey. We will identify possible obstacles that might hold you back. I will show you how you can push through resistance, though it might feel uncomfortable, or even impossible. You will learn that you alone hold the power you need to take full responsibility for your life. That is the only way.

We will look at goal-setting and decision making in a different way, allowing you to step into a future of your own making.

By doing these things, you will create the new and different future you crave.

I have been through this process. It was difficult for many different reasons. At the end of the day, though, I am much happier. I feel free and more in control of my own destiny.

Why I Wrote This Book

I am writing this book because I want you to learn from my experiences, making your own journey easier. I'm angry that so many health professionals are struggling to cope with the relentless pressure they are exposed to on a daily basis. Of course, we all work under stress and pressure at times, especially in the medical field. But if this pressure is balanced with calm periods, enough time away from work, and support, then that pressure is both acceptable and, for many doctors, part of the attraction of a medical career.

But the pendulum has swung too far to one side, and fundamental change is now needed. In the longer term, I do not believe that patients will be served by our sacrifice. The longer this continues, the more profound the collapse which now seems inevitable.

The fate of health care is at a critical stage in history. Modern technology and advances in treatment mean that an endless amount of money could be spent on research and development, as well as patient care, and still, it would not be enough. Modern societies will struggle more and more to fund the bottomless pit of health care. There needs to be a shift from *treating* ill health to *preventing* ill health.

This applies to patients, of course, but it also applies to you and to me.

Are you ready to make this change? Are you ready to put your own needs first? Lead by example? Living a joyful and healthy life is not just a pipe dream, it is absolutely possible.

So, let's get started.

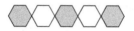

Chapter 1

My Story

Before we get stuck into the nitty-gritty of the book, I would like to tell you my own story.

Why I Chose to Be a Doctor

I grew up in a very small village in the south of Germany with my parents and an older brother. My father was absent most of the time; if not physically, then emotionally. My parents split up when I was 15, and I moved out with my mother and brother. I felt a lot of rejection from my father, and there was a big part of me that really wanted to please him, to get his approval.

The pressure to choose a certain career can be immense, and the reasons for this are external and internal. For me the main pressure was external, though this is not what it felt like. I felt I needed to impress and please my father to finally get his approval and love. Needless to say, most of this process was completely unconscious and only years later did I understand more about this internalized pressure.

I was the first doctor in my family, and it was a massive achievement for a girl growing up in a tiny village. Of course, it's a big achievement for anyone, as the work and commitment needed are immense.

But of course, as you might have guessed, me choosing to become a doctor did not yield the result I was craving. My father was proud of me, of course, but the emotional connection and love I was craving were not forthcoming. I now realize that this had nothing whatsoever to do with me, but purely with the person my father was. His own childhood had been traumatic and tough in many ways. Yet the course of my life took a completely different direction than it might otherwise have taken.

Even today I occasionally feel this urge to please him, and perhaps he symbolizes my need to receive external validation. This need was one of the factors that kept me locked into my career as a doctor for too long. The status and privileges that come with this role cannot be underestimated.

But I am not writing this book for him, nor to please anyone else I feel is an authority figure. I am writing this book for you and for me, to simply tell my story, share my experiences and what I have learned on my journey. This journey is uniquely individual and does not require justification, in the same way that *your* choices do not require justification. This book is unapologetic. Life needs to be unapologetic.

Picture Perfect, from the Outside Only

Thirty years later, I had a successful career as a family doctor. I was married with two children and a dog, my life busy and rewarding in so many ways.

Yet I did not feel happy.

Not only did I not feel happy, the strain and pressure of work were increasing with every passing year. Of course, this had something to do with the increasing workload that the caring professions experience in general, and working as a doctor will always be stressful and intense at times. But there was more going on than that.

If you looked at my life from the outside, it seemed perfect. Happy marriage, healthy children, successful career, no financial concerns, seemingly ideal.

I can tell you that it did not feel like this from the inside. I had no financial worries, but the psychological price I paid for that was high. My relationship with my husband was ok, but not as passionate and close as I would have loved it to be. I had no illness, but my diet was poor and I had neither motivation, nor the time or energy to embark on a regular exercise regime. I often snapped at my children since I simply did not have the mental and emotional energy at the end of a long day to give any more.

The worst part of that life was that I was feeling that stress but was unable to share it with anyone. Part of the medical professional persona is that we cope. That idea is drilled into medical students from day one. Patient care comes first, regardless of the pressures or cost to you.

Of course, patient care is crucial and my desire to help and contribute has not diminished over time. I have realized, though, that you cannot give from an empty cup.

Most mornings I would wake at 5 a.m. with anxiety and palpitations, the thought of what the day might bring already weighing heavy on my mind. The uncertainty and unpredictability of my job were getting more difficult to deal with. While at work I would cope, could never talk about what was really going on with me. How could I burden my colleagues, who were also struggling under the immense pressure I was under?

Slowly it began to dawn on me that I could not continue in this fashion. Something had to change. But it took years until I finally took the steps to change my life.

The problems I faced felt incredibly real and powerful: Concerns about letting my colleagues and patients down. Concerns about my financial future. Concerns about my pension. Concerns about what else I could do, what other career paths I could pursue. Perhaps it would be easier to just stick it out. Surely it isn't that bad after all.

But it was, and it got worse. I faced the option of burn-out, of not enjoying seeing patients anymore, of dreading every workday, of spending the weekend dreading the coming week; or making a change.

Reducing Pressure as a First Step

Even though I was not entirely sure what I was going to move towards, I realized I had to move away from the stress first. So my first step was to reduce my hours. I reduced my clinical commitment. I was still working almost a full-time week between different commitments, but I cut back on the most stressful aspect of my work.

I was lucky. I had a part-time administrative position, which provided me with some income while I was considering my options. I also had a plan, an idea of what I wanted to do instead. For me psychology, psychotherapy, hypnosis, and coaching had been a big interest for many years, and over that time I had spent quite a bit of time and money developing my skills in those areas.

I began to see clients for hypnosis and psychotherapy privately in addition to my clinical and administrative work. I loved having more time to spend with the people I worked with, being able to really get to the root of the problem and making real and effective changes in their lives. I would see people over six or eight weeks, identifying what was holding them back, and allowing them to face their fears in a supported environment without judgement. Sometimes only one session of intensive treatment was required to create lasting and profound change.

But then came the big change for me: I decided to leave my partnership. For weeks, I was agonizing about when and how to do it. More sleepless nights and anxiety attacks plagued me on a regular basis. Nothing significant happened to trigger my departure. I simply had enough of the relentless pressure at work.

A lot of thought and planning went into this final decision. I took a very close look at my finances to see how much money I needed to earn each month. I looked at ways to reduce my spending. For instance, I realized that I would no longer needed any childcare, as I would be able to plan my work around my children. I had the support of my husband and family. I knew that I could return to clinical medicine if things didn't work out. I did everything I could to make this step as easy and safe as possible. But despite all of my planning and caution, it was still agonizing. The thought of letting my family, my partners, and my patients down was overwhelming.

That day is vivid in my memory. My resignation letter clutched in my hands, I made my way to the senior partner's room, my heart pounding in my chest. I stood outside the door, considering whether this was really what I wanted to do. Years of hard work, a partnership I cherished, colleagues I respected, patients I had grown to love and really care for. Was I really ready to give it all up?

But the other side of the scale weighed heavier. It was my life at stake.

I knocked on the door and entered. I explained. I did not discuss the agony I had been feeling over such a long time, but my desire for a new life. A life of freedom and choice, of self-determination, of doing something I truly loved before it was too late. Even though I could see the shock in his face, my partner was incredibly understanding and supportive.

Of course, I did not know how this decision would unfold, but I had to trust that my feelings would not betray me. I still don't know where my final destination will be, but it will be of my making, a result of my choices.

Life Is Like a Recipe

I learned something important about life not that long ago. And it is quite simple.

There is a recipe for everything. Every feeling has a recipe. If I want to feel happy, I need to do things that make me happy, choose thoughts that make me happy, be in an environment that makes me happy. How can I expect to feel happy when I spend most of my time doing things I hate?

I realize that there are things that I need to do that will not make me ecstatically happy. But I can endeavor to do more of what makes me happy, less of what I dislike, and avoid the things I hate.

This is true for everything in life. Everything you experience is the effect or outcome of a recipe. By identifying what ingredients are required for your personal desired state, you can take control of the outcome. It is very much like baking. You simply do not expect to get a chocolate gateaux when your core ingredients are lemons. Lemons as ingredients might make a wonderful and refreshing piece of pastry, but part of a chocolate gateaux they are not. We cannot complain about what we have without being willing to change what ingredients go into creating the outcome.

We need to bring consciousness and awareness to what kind of life we want. Once we can take responsibility for our life, we reclaim the power to change and shape it according to our own decisions, even though this might feel scary, impossible, or downright selfish.

Priorities

My priorities were quite simple. Initially, it was a moving away from the intense feelings of stress and overwhelm, from not having any control over my working day. These stresses were spilling over into my everyday life, coloring everything with a dark hue.

I wanted to have more control over my life. I wanted to feel better, to be able to look forward to work, to feel free, light and joyful. I wanted to be able to spend more quality time with my children and husband. I wanted to be able to be more active, less exhausted and mentally drained.

I did not really know how I would accomplish all of this, but one thing was for sure: I wouldn't accomplish it by continuing to do the same thing over and over again.

As I moved away from what I didn't want, I began to see and create new opportunities, propelling me into a life I enjoy much more fully than I have for years.

Yes, I have less money now, but I have more freedom. Yes, there is still uncertainty and I sometimes wonder how everything will work out. I am still in the process of creating a life that more authentically reflects my values. This does not happen overnight—it's a process which is still ongoing. And no, I have not regretted my decision to leave.

I discovered the recipe for my own happiness. I am aware of the ingredients I need in my life to make me feel more fulfilled and much happier.

Life can still be scary, but it is also exciting, new, and fresh. It is a life of adventure and opportunity rather than drudgery and overwhelm.

The book will discuss the ingredients of my personal recipe for happiness, fulfillment and living an empowered life. The processes will be the same for you, though the ingredients you choose might be totally different.

I have helped many of my clients on this journey of identifying their passions and what is important to them, how to let go of outdated beliefs, heal old wounds, and create a life of freedom and choice. This is something you can achieve as well.

You will find all the necessary steps in this book, allowing you to bring clarity and awareness into the processes required to create a life you truly enjoy. This could mean stepping out of medicine for a while, changing your role, or perhaps doing something completely new that you haven't even considered yet. You will find the tools to make the right decision for you.

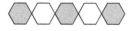

Chapter 2

The Costs of the Status Quo

The mind likes what is familiar. What is familiar is not necessarily the same as what would make us happy. I guess the reasons for this lie deep in our evolutionary history.

Physical survival is the number one priority of our mind. Thousands of years ago, wandering into unknown territory, accidentally meeting other tribes, or running into predatory animals could well have ended the lives of our ancestors. I am sure it did for quite a lot of them.

Despite the advances of humanity on so many levels, we still have our primitive brain which can have a powerful impact on our every action and behavior, often without conscious realization. Liking what is familiar aids our survival. If we are still alive, it means that whatever we have experienced has not killed us—yet, anyway. Part of our primitive brain, therefore, wants us to keep doing what we have always done.

We forget that that comes with a price, and that it can cost us our life over the longer term, and absolutely cost us the enjoyment of life today.

The Price Tag Principle

Everything in life has a price, a cost associated with it. The things we do and the things we don't do.

Ultimately, you are trading your life for what you do. The energy which is your life force goes into the things you do: your job, time spent with loved ones, time in nature, time to simply be, or whatever else you are pouring your energy into. We all know that this life does not go on forever. The life force, this specific life we have is limited. It will end sooner or later. So whatever it is we are trading our life for, it needs to be worth it.

Helping others certainly is worth a lot. Having the dedication to spend decades training, studying at great cost to yourself and your life, working unsocial hours, always putting others first, demonstrates the kind of person you are. I know how committed you are. I know how much you care. You have chosen this career for a reason, and I would like you to spend a few minutes now thinking about that reason. What were you hoping to gain from it? What was your pay off?

The cost of simply having gotten where you are is quite immense. There must have been a payoff, something that made it all worthwhile.

Perhaps it was the genuine need to help others. Perhaps you come from a family of doctors, and it was that pressure that persuaded you to pursue this career. Or you saw what a privilege it is to be able to work as a doctor. Perhaps it had to do with job security, status, and the privileges that come with being a physician. There are a multitude of reasons, and it is helpful to understand what motivated you.

It can be so easy to get dragged down a certain path and, before you know it, several decades have gone by and you suddenly realize that what you're doing is no longer servicing the debt, no longer enough to pay for your investment. The cost can become too high.

You may have been swept along by a powerful current like a leaf in a river, and it can be difficult to step out of this current. The momentum simply carries you forward, from one step to the next, year after year, until you realize your passion is gone, you are tired and drained, and there is nothing left for you to give.

This is your invitation to stop, pause and consider where this current is taking you. What will the ultimate price be for carrying on as you are? More importantly, are you willing to pay this price? Is the ultimate destination worth it?

Let's examine some of the likely costs if you change nothing.

The Cost to Your Health

I do not need to tell you how important health is. Without health, we have nothing. You see this every day at work. You see the suffering that poor health inflicts on people.

I am not simply talking about absence of disease. I am talking about how vibrant you feel; how much energy you have at your disposal to do the things you love. Is there a spring in your step and joy in your heart? Does your physical being, your body, support you in all the things you want to achieve?

I remember coming home after a long day at work, just barely able to muster the energy to have some sort of dinner, usually takeout, and then promptly fall asleep on the couch. I used to be exhausted and asleep before my young children would even be in their beds.

Health affects every area of your life. It affects how you feel. Your emotional life is hugely influenced by your health. It also affects your thinking and mental clarity. It affects how you see yourself and what you think you're able to achieve. It affects your character and your relationships. Being in pain or exhausted will have an impact on how you interact with your partner, children and loved ones. It will impact what you do daily.

Your health will affect your long-term plans. What are you planning to do when you finally retire? Will you be able to do these things without having taken care of your health in the meantime? We are talking about your long-term quality of life. About spending time with your grandchildren, traveling, or even just relaxing.

I was often too exhausted to even think about my long-term health or quality of life. I began to realize that I was no longer willing to pay with my health to satisfy the strains and stresses of the daily grind.

Being healthy is generally simple, provided you are not suffering from any illness or disease. Exercise, enough rest, and the right diet. A balanced life. We all know the right things to do, but whether we do them is a different thing altogether.

Doctors are in a terrible bind. We know the healthy things to do, but often do not have the energy, time, or will to do them. If you are like me, you believe you should be able to manage it all; you should know everything, cope with everything, and find it difficult to ask for help. This thinking can leave you feeling isolated and helpless. This thinking can leave you feeling guilty and disempowered.

A colleague of mine suffered from an eating disorder as a teenager. She made a good recovery, but this recovery depends on her being able to manage her stress levels, to have enough energy and time to consider her meal plan and cook healthy and nutritious foods. This challenge is huge, and often she is left feeling overwhelmed with the intensity and stress of her work. It will come to no surprise to you that she reverts to binge eating as a way of coping. She is sacrificing her own needs, her own health, to remain in a system which is incredibly damaging.

We all have different coping strategies, but none address the real underlying issues—they only sugar coat things. We are papering over the cracks, suffering alone until we simply can't keep up the act anymore.

If you believe you can work in this way in the longer term, not looking after yourself as well as you could, without any consequences, you might need to reconsider your position.

Chronic Stress

Before looking at the impact of this work on your relationships, let's spend a little time looking at chronic stress. I am acutely aware that I am not telling you anything new, but please bear with me as I remind you what chronic stress does to the body.

Chronic stress levels lead to raised cortisol levels for prolonged periods of time, and this can cause significant damage to the body, brain, and mind. Brain structure, brain size, and function all change if you are exposed to chronic stress, down to a genetic level.

Though there are several body systems which are responsible for these reactions, the starting point is the amygdala, part of the limbic system, situated deep within the brain. This is our fear center.

If exposed to chronic stress, this structure increases both its activity level and neural connections. At the same time the function of the hippocampus, also a part of the limbic system, deteriorates. The hippocampus is responsible for learning, memory and stress control. In other words, the more stressed you are, the less able to *deal with* this stress you are.

The limbic system plays a key part in the regulation of emotions, and the amygdala has been linked to both fear responses and pleasure. Your perception of fear and pleasure changes, more things appear overwhelming, and fewer things are able to make you feel happy.

Being exposed to too much cortisol over a prolonged time leads to the loss of neural connections and shrinks the brain overall. In addition to this it can cause the pre-frontal cortex to shrink. This part of the brain has been called our "genius." It is important for concentration, decision making, judgement and social interactions. This might well be the reason why our decision-making processes can be impaired when we are under intense stress or overly fearful.

Being overly stressed or fearful over a prolonged period will also have a detrimental effect on the functioning of memory. We might become forgetful. The learning of new knowledge or skills can be difficult.

As a doctor, your life can be extremely stressful. The pressures you face daily can be immense. Interestingly, our bodies react to stress in the same way, regardless of whether the threat is real or imagined. This was particularly pertinent for me when I was spending my mornings worrying about what work would be like, really imagining it, feeling it, and dreading it. It seems that this alone can be damaging, regardless of whether work itself was manageable in the end or not.

These stress hormones put us into survival mode, searching for outside threats and solutions. With this, our focus also moves to the outside world to the detriment of our inner experiences. This is when we are at risk of losing touch with ourselves, our yearning, our ambitions, and our passion.

We lose touch with our inner peace, quiet, and serenity as our minds keep looking out for threats. Once this condition becomes chronic, our health can suffer in a myriad of ways. We live in a modern society with fewer real threats requiring an intense physiological reaction such as the fight or flight reaction, yet we still have our ancient brain reacting as though we do.

Many people live in chronic states of stress, unhappiness, anxiety, and depression. I know. I saw it in many of my patients and my colleagues. I saw it in myself.

Burn-Out

Chronic stress leads to burn-out. Studies have found that a significant percentage of family doctors suffer from burn-out. Studies have also shown that this burn-out did not necessarily impact patient safety or quality of care. But how does it impact the quality of life for the doctor concerned? What does it mean for the self-image and expectation the doctor has of herself?

Not long before I made the decision to leave my practice, I remember a patient coming to see me. As it happened on a frequent basis, the patient entered the room, sat down, and burst into tears. It took her a minute before she was even able to verbalize what upset her so much. At that moment, instead of feeling empathy and compassion for a distressed human being, my inner dialogue said something completely different. It went along the lines of: "Oh my God, I do not have time for this. I wonder how many patients are waiting already; I am already running late; how will I ever catch up? When will I find the time to look at my results and write my referrals? I just can't deal with this right now."

I caught myself thinking this and was horrified. Chronic stress had turned me into a person lacking in compassion, more and more focused on my own survival.

For so long, I did not even allow myself to acknowledge these thoughts. Was I the only one thinking this? The only one feeling emotionally overwhelmed and drained while at the same time beating myself up for not being superhuman?

Reality check: I am only human. You are only human. We are people like all others, with emotions, fears, concerns, and a limited amount of energy. And yes, we can make mistakes. Yet doctors are expected to work and function perfectly in an increasingly pressured environment, where the stakes are extremely high.

Fear of Consequences

Lives are at stake. The lives of our patients. Every decision you make can have serious consequences. Fear of mistakes, fear of complaints, fear of being sued are part of the reality of many health professionals.

Complaints can be absolutely devastating.

Many years ago, I received a complaint that still haunts me. I remember my practice manager approached me in the corridor, his face expressing concern. A complaint had been made against me, a patient demanding money—otherwise she would take things further.

My heart seemed to stop. It felt as though an icy fist had reached into my chest and was squeezing hard. The walls were closing in as the sense of devastation, panic, and fear were getting overwhelming. I felt frozen into a state of anxiety and fear, unable to move on.

We looked at the notes and the complaint together. The patient had a condition I had considered during the consultation, yet thought it unlikely that she had it. It turned out I was wrong. The patient needed surgery and, thankfully, made a full recovery. She suffered more than was necessary. The operation was unavoidable, but it could have been better planned with an earlier diagnosis.

I was so very sorry that I had not picked it up, even though I had considered the condition. I had made my decision based on clinical findings. Medicine is a hard science, but in practice it is also an art. Every day brings a multitude of opportunities to get it wrong, to make mistakes.

Though the complaint went no further, it stayed with me for a long time. The emotional impact it had was devastating. The uncertainty and fear of what else might happen impacted every aspect of my life. There was not a minute in the day I did not think about it. There were times I was crying so much I had to hide from my children. The medicine I was practicing became more defensive, subjecting patients to unnecessary investigations and referrals. No one benefits from that defensiveness.

For me this was a turning point.

Impact on Relationships

After that episode with the complaint, I realized that continuing long term in medicine was not an option. I was not going to be that person. I was changing, my personality was changing, I felt forced into survival mode. I was not prepared to pay this price, it was simply too high.

The impact of chronic stress on our relationships is significant. Not only relationships with patients, but also our closest family, children, and friends.

Apart from being short with my children at times and not having enough energy to do things together, my work left me too exhausted to cook good quality food for them. Cooking was always the first thing to go when I got stressed and overwhelmed. The guilt I felt about that was not insignificant.

Of course, other relationships can suffer too. Not many of my friends are doctors. With them, I found myself unable to fully share the stresses I faced and their impact on my life and my being. No one who has not worked under these pressures can fully understand the impact it has.

For many doctors this can be very isolating. Human beings are social animals, and connection to a tribe and a sense of belonging is crucial when it comes to our well-being on all levels.

The need to belong is a very powerful human need. Not fulfilling that need is the cause of much suffering and pain in the world. Quite naturally we want to stay close to the people who we believe truly understand us, understand the pressure and stress, and who can also share our victories and successes. The medical community is such a community, perhaps in a similar way that army veterans feel very strongly about the brotherhood they experience as part of their unit.

I wonder, though, how healthy and helpful it is to remain so closely linked to a group that sees things very black and white, whose expectations are based on a very traditional model of acting, thinking, and being.

Overall, I have felt supported by the doctors around me. As work pressures rise, the compassion amongst the teams gets more and more strained. There is always the expectation to go to work, regardless of how you feel. Everyone knows how much greater the pressure on the team becomes if just one person is off sick.

I used to worry about getting to work to find one of my colleagues was out that day for whatever reason. The feeling of overwhelm and dread so intense, the sense of disempowerment so great, that I often wondered how other people could cope with this relentless pressure. How are you coping? How long do you think you will be able to cope? And at what cost?

Life Expectancy

One frequently quoted study on life expectancy talks about head teachers and their significantly reduced life expectancy if they retire at 65 instead of 60 years of age. This suggests that having a highly stressful job later in life significantly reduces the length of life. I can't comment on the validity of this study, but I can say that these findings make sense to me.

At the same time, there is no denying that professional people tend to have a higher life expectancy overall, and that general life expectancy continues to increase.

As the retirement age continues to increase, these are serious considerations. How long do you think will you be able to continue to work like you do? Will it be safe? Will you be able to keep up with the ever-changing knowledge and technology flooding the profession?

Of course, life expectancy is important, but one could argue that quality of life is even more important than the length of life.

Quality of Life

The price of your quality of life is perhaps the highest to pay on a day-to-day basis.

Let's consider some essential questions before moving on.

What is the purpose of this life anyway?

What are you hoping to get out of it?

What do you want to add and contribute to the world?

What do you want to experience in your life?

The answers to these questions are deeply personal, and we will explore these issues in much more depth later.

For now, let us simply consider what your daily quality of life is like. Are you happy? Do you wake up, eager to jump out of bed, looking forward to the day ahead? Is there joy in your heart and in your step?

Or do you feel the way I felt for much too long: exhausted, waking at 5 a.m. with anxiety, dreading the day, and looking forward to the end of the working week, only to spend the weekend worrying about the beginning of the next working week?

There were many things I loved about my work. I loved spending time with patients, being part of a team, the challenge of dealing with undifferentiated illness. But these aspects of my work became more and more overshadowed by the relentless pressure and increasing workload.

I simply did not enjoy life much anymore. I was tired, I forgot what I felt passionate about, and ultimately, I realized that something had to change.

Regrets at the End of Life

Like me, you probably see many patients coming to the end of their lives. Have any of these patients ever expressed regret at not having spent more time at work?

In my experience accompanying patients during this time of their lives, I discovered there were several common regrets they had, which are not that surprising.

Most of my patients wished they had had the courage to live a more authentic life, a life determined by their own choices, dreams and ambitions; not a life expected of them by others. They wished they had spent less time at work. They wished they had expressed their feelings more and allowed themselves to be happy, rather than trying to fit in a box and conforming to societal norms and expectations. They discovered that happiness is a choice, in the same way that fulfilling your dreams and aspirations is a choice.

Ultimately, people wished they could have lived an authentic life, a life fitting to themselves, their wishes, their desires and passions. This is not necessarily an easy life, but a life that is self-determined, lived with courage and conviction. A life worth remembering as you look back over it. It was this impetus that led me to make these huge changes in my life. I did not want to get to the end of my life and have the same regrets that many of my patients had. I would rather take a risk and fail than never have tried at all.

EXERCISE:
COSTS AND BENEFITS

We have looked in some detail at the possible costs of continuing to work the way you do. It is crucial for you to really understand the impact, both for your immediate quality of life and in the longer term.

Here is a simple yet powerful exercise that allows you to see some pros and cons of making a change.

Step one: Write down all the benefits of continuing as you are. These could be related to your finances, job security, team working, and anything else you can think of.

Step two: Write down the cost that comes with not changing anything. What is the cost to your relationships, your health, your emotional, mental and spiritual well-being? How about your overall quality of life, your dreams, and aspirations?

Step three: Write down the possible benefits should you decide to make a change. What could your life look like? How would you like to work, what would you like to be or do? What would you gain? What is your life vision? What would living an authentic life look like for you? Allow yourself to freely imagine and feel what this life could be like.

Once you have completed all three parts, take a moment to look at your answers. On the left side you have the answers to question one, and on the right the answers to questions two and three.

The result of this simple exercise gives you a clue as to where you need to focus your efforts. If the list on the left is longer than the one on the right, it is likely that the benefits of your current clinical practice outweigh any possible gain arising from a change. In this case, it might be best to address single pain points and focus on improving your working conditions, making your life less stressful and more fulfilling.

If the list on the right is longer, it might be worthwhile to consider a more radical solution. This means that you might benefit from leaving your current position, and it is certainly worthwhile to explore a variety of options.

I am curious about what you have written. I would love to know your thoughts and discuss this with you. I truly believe that a new and better life is possible for you, regardless of whether you choose to stay or leave.

Key Points to Take Away

This chapter explored the possible costs you might face if you do not change the direction of your life. We spoke about the price tag principle and the effects of your working conditions on every aspect of your life: the impact on your relationships, your health, and your overall quality of life. As health professionals, we all face the possibility of burn-out as the chronic stress takes its toll. We discussed possible regrets many people face at the end of their lives.

And we began to look at pros and cons of staying as you are, or making a change into a life more in alignment with your values and priorities.

In the next chapter, we are going to look in much more detail at the tools you need to make the transition into a new and more empowered life, a life of your making, should you choose to take this step.

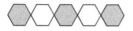

Chapter 3

Tools

The first step on every journey must be to figure out the destination. Without this you simply cannot get there. No doubt you will get somewhere, but it could be anywhere. If anywhere is fine for you, you can carry on as you are, but if you want to have any chance of achieving the life you desire, you need to define what that life looks like first. And don't worry, you can change your mind along the way at any point.

To figure this out we are going to do an exercise. Most of the exercises in this book are quite simple, but do not be fooled by their simplicity. Firstly, simple does not equal easy, and secondly, it is the simple things that often have the most profound impact.

———————— **EXERCISE:** ————————
WHAT DO I REALLY WANT?
HOW DO I WANT TO FEEL?

It can be quite difficult to verbalize your desires, to have clarity about what you truly want.

Most people never really think deeply enough about this. Sometimes the chronic stress and pressures of daily life can cut you off from the part of you that knows. It is, therefore, easier sometimes to start with what you do **not** want.

There are several steps in this process, and we will begin by identifying what you no longer want in your life. Make a list of all these things. Be very specific.

It is not enough to say: "I do not want to be unhappy or stressed." You need to say what exactly it is that makes you unhappy or stressed. One example might be: "I no longer want to work in such a busy and stressful environment that I come home too exhausted to spend any time with my children." Or it could be: "I no longer want to be on-call on my own, having to deal with all emergencies without support." The more specific you can be, the better.

Next, make a list of the things you want instead of this first list. Simply take each point and rephrase it into what you want, rather than what you don't want. This forces you to put what you want into a positive context, rather than a negative one.

For the examples I gave this could be: "I want to work in an environment that is both stimulating and motivates me, leaves me energized and capable of having a fulfilled home life." And "I want to work in a team with clearly defined support for the doctor on call."

As you do this, new questions might arise. What would this work environment look like? What is it that you find both stimulating and motivating? How can you change your current work situation to reflect this better? This is not an exercise to find out whether these things are possible or not. I want you to do this exercise as if you had a magic wand, and with a simple swish you could have all that you desired.

Take your time to do this exercise. It is very important that you are clear about what you do and do not want, as specifically as possible.

After having completed the first two parts of the exercise, the third part is to identify what you want that is not the opposite of what you don't want. In other words, what else do you want in your life?

So, make a list of all the other things you would like to have in your life. It is very important not to censor this. Do not leave anything out because you think it might not be possible to achieve it anyway.

You might be surprised what you come up with. Perhaps a childhood dream of having a dog, perhaps the wish to travel the world. Perhaps you always wanted to work as a piano teacher when you were a child. It could be anything at all.

I want you to consider other career choices as well. What were you passionate about as a child, between the ages of 7 and 14? What fascinated you? What did you spend most of your time doing? This can give you vital clues. If you could no longer be a doctor, what else would you love to be or do? It could be anything at all.

This first step is crucial; once you have done this exercise you will know what you do and do not want. Later, we will discuss how to use this knowledge to begin to create a life much more in alignment with your desires.

Another crucial part of this exercise is to identify how you want to feel.

The Power of Emotions

Emotions are incredibly powerful. They are the reason we do anything at all. For example, we don't go on vacation just to be away from home. What would be the point of that? We go on vacation because it makes us feel a certain way. It can make you feel free and joyful. It can make you feel warm, especially if you normally live in Scotland, like I do. Or it can bring excitement into your life, depending on your destination and chosen activities.

We don't own a certain car, or home, or anything else just because we can, but because it makes us feel a certain way.

Most of us like to feel positive. This could mean feeling happy, connected, powerful, loved, cherished, or important. There is a myriad of ways we describe the specific feelings, but they tend to be on a higher vibration rather than a lower vibration. Feelings on a lower vibration could be doubt, fear, anxiety, or concern.

The point here is that we seek out certain emotions and try to avoid others. How we feel about anything is what colors our life, makes it worthwhile or utterly miserable.

All feelings are normal, and it is not the feeling itself but the *meaning* we give to the feeling that makes all the difference. We tend to identify with our feelings rather than use them in a constructive way. We tend to think that we have no control over how we feel, that our feelings just happen. Neither approach is true or particularly helpful.

Why do we have feelings anyway? What is the point of them?

I found it always quite strange to think that here I am, only one small person among billions on Earth, hurtling on this rock through space at tremendous speed in an infinitely large universe, and the fact that a patient shouted at me can ruin my whole day. Why would I even care about something as trivial as that?

Feelings can simply be so overwhelming, so powerful and intense, that we forget everything else. They take us on a ride, and unless we can take control it is very difficult to get off.

In my opinion, the real purpose of feelings is to act as signposts. They are signals allowing us to identify whether we are moving in a positive direction. This does not mean, necessarily, that a positive feeling equals a positive direction. If only it was that simple. Sometimes it is the resistance and the pain that signals a positive direction.

This is where the growth lies, the growing edge of our personal evolution, and like all growth, it can be painful. Feelings are a call to action, they invite us to look deeper.

I wonder: Which are the feelings you are seeking? Which are the feelings you are seeking to avoid? What does this tell you about yourself as a person?

Personally, I always sought to avoid conflict. I would rather sacrifice my own desires and needs than to stand up and fight for myself, or even say what I wanted. The pain of doing this has finally outweighed the potential benefit, and though my journey has been filled with doubt and fear, I realized this was the path I had to tread.

This is the path that leads to the authentically positive feelings, rather than those gained through avoidance and self-sacrifice. It leads to the feelings we all yearn for.

This journey of transformation you are on can be painful and difficult in so many ways, but just the fact that you are feeling like this does not mean you are wrong to embark on this journey. You are not alone, I will journey with you; my voice will accompany you every step of the way.

Identifying Passions and Values

At this stage, you will have a better understanding of what it is that you do and do not want as well as the feelings you are seeking. The next step is to identify where this is leading you.

You know that something needs to change, otherwise you would not be reading this book. Things are not great at work. Perhaps you are not clear yet what this change will entail. Will it simply mean a restructuring of your working day, moving to a different position, or leaving medicine altogether?

Identifying your passions and values can help you to make this decision. It is crucial that your passions, values, and daily activities are in alignment. When they are not we begin to feel unhappy and uncentered.

There are only three things which drive human behavior: your beliefs and paradigms, what you believe to be true about yourself and the world; your habits, the things you do on a day to day basis; and your values. Your values can be a powerful motivator to carry you through very tough times, to make difficult decisions, but only if your belief system, your daily habits, and values are in alignment.

Let me illustrate this to you. Most doctors value patient care very highly. I know you do, otherwise you would not be reading this book. Patient-centered care, the desire to alleviate suffering, is a value that you hold close to your heart. But it is very likely that the pressures at work and the sheer volume and complexity of your workload do not allow you to fully bring this value into your working day. In other words, you do not have the time that would truly be needed to address your patient's needs thoroughly and with compassion. If this happens on occasion you can cope well, but if it happens day after day and month after month, there comes a point when you begin to feel very unsatisfied with your work. Your values, daily habits, and belief system are not aligned.

Eventually one of two things will happen: you must either change what you do to get back into alignment with your values, or give up on your values to fit into the existing structure.

There are no easy answers. But I know that the first option allows you to continue to live as an empowered and authentic being, and the other leads you down a path of disempowerment, of feeling resentful and embittered, of burn-out.

It can be extremely helpful to get back in touch with your values and passions, so, before we move on, I would like you to spend a little bit of time doing just that. Remember that I asked you the reasons you became a doctor in the first place? These reasons are your passions and the values you hold dear.

Identifying Priorities

No one value is better or worse than another. We have different values because we are different people. It is likely that you have a variety of different values and passions.

Let me give you some examples of values that might appeal to you: kindness, justice, service, compassion, nurturing, and warmth. There are many others which are also likely to be important to you, such as abundance, accomplishment, knowledge, friendship. Or maybe success, loyalty, playfulness, adventure.

To make a decision that is right for you, you must find out which of the values you hold are the most important for you. There is no judgement here, but you can see that someone whose priority is abundance will make a different decision from a person who holds compassion as their highest value, in the same way that adventure would lead you down a different path than loyalty.

Spend a few minutes and make a list of 10–15 values and then circle the top 3–5. Put them in order and you will have your top 3–5 values.

Once you have identified these, they must play an important part in your decision making. Allowing your values to aid you in your decision-making means that you have the knowledge and understanding of where you are headed. It enables you to not only make empowered decisions but to have the confidence of knowing where the path will lead. You will not necessarily know the how, but you will know the what and where.

Of course, putting your values first and using them as the basis for your decision-making will mean that some of these decisions will be tough and very likely life-changing. It will mean that others might not agree with your choices since their values and priorities are different from yours. Ultimately though, it is only through this process that you will reach alignment between your values and the life you live.

Confidence

I could assume that you are confident. You are a doctor, after all. You work in a high-pressured job, must make a multitude of decisions every day, and deal with very difficult situations, patients, and possibly colleagues.

I will not make this assumption though. I am sure you are confident in many areas of your life and career, yet there is still a part of you that is unsure. This part which just wants things to be ok, just wants to be able to get on with the job you love; if only you could, all would be well.

But you cannot. You would not be reading this book if you could. The system you find yourself in does not allow this. The system forces you to work under immense pressure, meanwhile telling you that there is something wrong with you if you cannot take it.

Over time, this can erode your confidence significantly. You are so busy that there is no time to reflect. There is no time to consider your options. There is no time to fully understand that pursuing what you seek, following your values and empowering yourself will also empower your patients and ultimately improve the system significantly.

This change will be painful for all involved, including your patients. This is certainly one reason that can hold you back, and we will discuss this and other reasons in more detail in the next chapter.

For now, let me simply emphasize the importance of being confident. Confident in the validity of your values, confident in your right to live a life in alignment with these values, and confident in your ability to make all the changes necessary to bring this about.

Self-Compassion

One crucial piece of this puzzle of confidence is self-compassion. Compassion is very important when it comes to patient care. We all understand this clearly.

Compassion is a feeling of distress for the suffering of others, often including the desire to alleviate this suffering.

You could argue that too much compassion for others makes it very difficult to sustain a career in the caring professions for a whole lifetime, as the emotional strain of constantly doing this is immense. Self-compassion can certainly be a lifeline during this journey.

Unfortunately, it has been my experience that self-compassion is in short supply within the medical profession. I have experienced this personally, with a lack of compassion for myself, and also have seen it in most of my colleagues.

We tend to be harsh and critical with ourselves, always striving for perfection. We have a need to know everything and control everything. We have already spoken about the fear of making mistakes and the horror this can wreak within our lives. Mistakes are meant to be discussed in blame-free culture, but I know that that frequently doesn't happen. Sometimes we are blamed by colleagues, and sometimes by patients. Even if others do not blame us, we tend to blame ourselves.

By the nature of our jobs we can deal with very unwell people. Despite what medicine can offer, and despite all the medical advances in recent years, often our patients still deteriorate and die. To come to terms with witnessing the distress of our patients and their families, often helpless to change the outcome, is not an easy feat. To have a healthy amount of self-compassion is crucial in this context. After all, we are human, we have feelings, we get tired, we can make mistakes, we are not perfect, yet are expected to always get it right.

So, what exactly is self-compassion? Self-compassion is to bestow compassion on our own selves, especially when we perceive ourselves to be inadequate in any way, when we have failed, made a mistake, are not as successful or smart as we think we ought to be.

The crux here is to show compassion in the face of perceived inadequacy. Yet it is exactly this inadequacy that we seek to avoid at all cost, as the cost of inadequacy in the medical field can be extremely high, both in financial and emotional terms.

Despite all of this we all need to cultivate self-compassion. We need to move away from shame, blame, and guilt.

Shame, Blame and Guilt

These feelings undermine what we do; they undermine our personality, change how we practice, change how we interact with patients, and color everything in our lives with or without our conscious awareness. They destroy our quality of life. And most importantly, they are not good for patient care, the very thing you are likely to hold dearest to your heart.

We get so used to feeling like this that we forget that it does not have to be this way. Remember the joy and bliss you felt before this heavy burden was placed on your shoulders? I have glimpses of the joyous and free feeling I used to have in a life before taking on all this responsibility.

I realize that this will not happen overnight, but unless we begin to move into that direction, it will not happen at all.

I would like you to spend a little bit of time every day practicing kindness for yourself. This is best done first thing in the morning before you even get out of bed, or last thing at night, before you close your eyes. Regard yourself and your decisions with compassion, with forgiveness, with love. Regard yourself as you would your best friend, your partner, or your child.

It might feel uncomfortable to do this, it might be unfamiliar. Remember the beginning of the second chapter? The mind likes what is familiar. The key here is that you can make anything you choose familiar, simply by doing it on a regular basis. Before long, this new behavior becomes normal.

It depends on what you want in your life, which values you wish to integrate and how you want to feel. You know this now, you have completed the exercises, all that is required now is to identify what steps you need to take to make it happen and bring it into your life.

Mindfulness

An essential tool in your arsenal is mindfulness. It is very popular now, and there are a significant number of studies out there demonstrating the benefits of being mindful. It is associated with better mood, improved sleep, and less anxiety.

For me, mindfulness is very much about living in the now. Not thinking about what happened in the past or worrying about what might happen in the future. Spending too much time thinking about the past is associated with depression, and too much time spent anticipating a certain future is linked with anxiety. Of course, this does not mean that both past and future do not deserve thought and attention—of course they do. But an excessive amount of time spent doing that is unhealthy.

How do you know how much is healthy in this context? I would suggest that when you no longer enjoy what you are doing now because your thoughts are with the past or future, if you find that you need to drag your attention back to the now, if you struggle to fall asleep because your mind is too active, then you need to be more mindful.

The human mind is truly amazing: not bound by time or matter, but free to venture anywhere and anytime. The danger is that this can lead us to being ungrounded, not in touch with our body and our senses, disconnected from reality, and firmly encased in a mental construct of our own making.

The solution is both simple and beautiful. Just return your full conscious awareness to your senses. What do you see right now? Pay attention to the colors, the shapes, the shadows of what you observe. Be like a child who sees this for the very first time. What can you hear? Is there silence? The rustling of the wind in the trees? Or perhaps there is noise. What can you smell or taste? And what do you feel? What does your body feel like? Is there tension in your neck, perhaps an ache or discomfort somewhere? Spend a few moments scanning your body and allow it to move of its own volition.

Focus on your breath, becoming aware of the air flowing in and out of your body. Feeling the temperature of the air as it travels through your nostrils, the rise and fall of your abdomen. These things bring you back to the here and now. Every time you feel stressed or your thoughts run away with you, bring yourself back to the eternal now.

These are exercises which, despite their simplicity, have the most powerful impact on all the clients I work with. As I guide my clients through the steps allowing them to become masterful at these skills, they realize that they can always handle what is happening in the now.

In truth, now is all we have. There is no other time. You can remember the past, but you remember it in the now, you can never go back other than in your thoughts. Even if you think you have the same emotions and fears or concerns, they are only the emotions, fears, and concerns you are creating right now, not then. You can think about and plan the future, but again, you do this in the now; thinking about it will not take you there.

How to Deal with Overwhelm

I am aware of how overwhelming life can get.

I remember a little cartoon a friend of mine had up on her wall. It showed a little man, struggling under the weight of heavy bags. He said, "Usually I deal with one day at a time, but recently several days have tried to attack me all at once!"

I loved this little cartoon. We can always cope with one thing at a time, but if too many things need our attention all at once, it becomes too much very quickly. Being mindful and simply doing one thing at a time will help with this feeling of overwhelm.

We have all been there: the phone rings, a patient sits in front of you, and a nurse is at your door, rushing in as the patient leaves and asking her question before you even had the chance to finish writing up your notes. These days, I stop her, saying that my aging brain can only do one thing at a time, and could she please wait until I have finished with my notes.

Key Points to Take Away

At the end of this chapter you will have so much more clarity as to exactly what it is that you want and the values you hold closest to your heart. We have explored the power of emotions and understand how overwhelming they can be, but now we also understand their true purpose as signposts. Even feelings of resistance and anxiety can affirm we are on the right path.

The clarity and awareness you have gained will be crucial in helping you come to the right decision for your own life in due course.

We explored the importance of confidence in your goals and the value of self-compassion and mindfulness.

These are all tools that will be of great assistance as you embark on this journey of decision making. Like any journey, there will be obstacles, certain beliefs and structures that can get in your way. This is what we will be exploring in the next chapter.

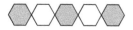

Chapter 4

Identifying the Obstacles

If moving into a more stress-free and joyous life was easy, you would not be reading this book. You know things need to change, but you feel stuck. You feel that either the system or yourself keeps you locked into place, unable to break free.

There are several reasons that can keep us all stuck, and they seem incredibly powerful and real to us.

The BIG Why

In the last chapter, we discussed the importance of values in the process of your decision making. Values are so important because they give us the *why* of all our decisions. You have identified what you want and how you want to feel in an ideal world, but unless you have a strong enough reason or purpose, relatively small obstacles will be able to derail you.

The why gives you the motivation to do what is necessary to get where you want to go. Let's explore this a little more deeply.

Let's say you had to train for a marathon. You have six months to get fit, but every day, as you are due to practice, you find a reason why you can't. It's raining, it's too cold, you feel tired, you need to do the grocery shopping. The list of reasons *not* to do it is endless. You clearly do not have a big enough reason to achieve your goal, otherwise these small things wouldn't stop you.

Let's say that your best friend tells you that he will take you on an exotic vacation to a place you have always wanted to visit, but only if you successfully train for and complete the marathon. This might increase your motivation and make it more likely for you to achieve your goal. But what if I told you the only way you will ever see your best friend again is to successfully train for and complete this marathon? Your motivation would be even higher. Suddenly there is a reason, such a compelling reason for you to accomplish your goal, that no obstacle could get in your way.

This is why your values are so important, this is why the purpose of what you are trying to achieve needs to be crystal clear in your mind. This purpose allows you to overcome any obstacle. I would like you to keep this reason in mind as we look at possible obstacles.

Just like it is important to identify and have clarity about what you want, it is also crucial to understand what can get in your way or hold you back. This is what this chapter is all about.

It is likely that the exploration of these issues will take you out of your comfort zone. That's good.

> *"A comfort zone is a beautiful place, but nothing ever grows there."*
> **Jane Travis**

Own Where You Are

The very first thing to do is to honestly acknowledge where you are in terms of your career and your life in general. Any form of sugar-coating, denial, or self-deception won't help you here.

There is a beautiful quote I heard some time ago, but unfortunately can't remember who said it. It goes along the lines of, "In order to leave a place you first need to arrive there." In other words, unless you honestly acknowledge the reality of the situation you are in and how you feel about it, you will remain stuck there. It can be painful to acknowledge this place, as it brings up issues around our identity and self-image. It can bring into stark contrast who we would like to be, who we see ourselves to be, how much we can cope with, and the reality of the situation.

To arrive where you're at, you will need the tools we discussed in the last chapter: self-compassion, kindness, and mindfulness. Simply acknowledging where you are without judgement is incredibly powerful.

The Importance of Meaning

The meaning we give to everything in our lives is part of what keeps us stuck. This might be the biggest obstacle of them all.

The human mind is a meaning making machine.

Let's think of an example. A young child, let's say a boy, has a busy mother who works several jobs to provide all the essentials for her family. When Mom gets home she is exhausted and all she wants is some quiet time.

Every time the boy comes up to Mom after work, she tells him to go away and do something else. Now, what conclusion do you think the child will draw from these events? In other words, what meaning will he attribute to what is happening?

Most likely the boy will think, "I am not important to my mom, something else always comes first." Now, this won't happen if this is a rare event, but if it happens often enough the child will conclude, "I am not important."

From the child's point of view, this meaning was the logical conclusion. It's unlikely that a young child has the life experience and wisdom to realize that this is not necessarily the truth. It might be true, but there are many reasons or meanings for an event like this. In this case, the real reason is that Mom is tired working several jobs and does not have the energy to devote to her child when she comes home from work. But for the child, the meaning of not being important becomes associated with this event, and any future events will consolidate this thinking further.

For the boy, this meaning becomes a truth. "I am not important" becomes a statement of fact, and could have a profound impact on everything in his life, from jobs to relationships, from the ability to experience joy to setting goals in his life.

But can you see that this isn't the truth, but simply a wrong meaning given to a recurring event? Sadly, for the child, that meaning often remains the truth unless somebody is able to convince him otherwise.

What does this mean for us? It means that we give meaning to everything that happens in our life. We judge things. Something is either good or bad, right or wrong, painful or pleasurable. We judge what we observe in others, see on TV, online, or in the newspaper. Sometimes, of course, we simply adopt the meaning that others have given to what's going on. The problem is that we believe that this meaning is inherent in the thing or event we observe or experience. They seem to be inextricably linked to each other, as well as being independent of us. This in turn means that there is nothing we can do about the meaning of anything. This point of view is totally disempowering, but we often don't realize that we are the ones creating the meaning.

Not only do we give meaning to things, we often believe that the meaning we have attributed to the event is the only possible explanation. Any similar future events are given the same meaning. In other words, we link events and similar events to the same meaning, and this link is very powerful.

In the brain the same nerve fibers are fired every time we give the same meaning to similar events, strengthening that association. In the end, the pattern that evolves is so strong that it can seem that the meaning we give to the event is the only possible meaning.

Let's question this premise, as it's not a fact. The meaning we have given to an event or experience is very often not the truth, but only one possible explanation for the situation.

Events have no meaning until we give them meaning. And this means we have a choice.

Fear of Being Judged

Most people attribute meaning to things in the way we have just discussed. This means that whatever you do or don't do will stimulate this process in your loved ones, friends, and colleagues. In other words, there will be judgement.

Other people will interpret your actions within the framework of their own beliefs. Of course, this judgement has nothing to do with you as such, but with the person doing the judging. Even so, the perceived pressure is immense. Our need to belong is very strong indeed, and stepping away from the norm, making a choice that is not perceived as "the done thing" requires courage and conviction. The more out with the norm we step, the harsher the judgement can be.

You might be surprised, though, how many people secretly admire your courage to step into a better life. They might wish they could do the same, but they allow the obstacles they face to hold them back.

We can decide not to attribute meaning to events, but simply observe the facts as they are. We can decide not to worry about how others attribute meaning to what we do, in the knowledge that this is merely a reflection of their own patterns that has nothing to do with us.

Staying open to the possibility of different meanings is empowering. It offers choice and the opportunity to question what is really happening, and it stops us from forming false, unhelpful, or damaging beliefs.

Fear of Change

"This is all very interesting," you might say, "but what does it have to do with my problem?"

It has everything to do with your problem. We tend to cling to the meaning we give to what is going on in our lives. We do this for the simple reason that it makes us feel more secure. It gives us stability. It gives predictability to a life which we fear might be just the opposite, unstable and unpredictable. We do this even if it keeps us stuck in a bad situation.

The meanings we give to everything and the resulting beliefs create the walls of the mental prison we erect for ourselves. If we realized that it was us who were responsible for this in the first place, that meaning and event are not the same, we would have the power to change this easily. But it is not so easy. We struggle to see the walls of this prison. It does not matter how often we redecorate our prison cell, as long as the walls are still standing, we remain trapped.

I have often wondered why women can stay so long in abusive relationships. Of course, this is a difficult problem with many layers of complexity and no easy answer. There is no "one size fits all" answer. But perhaps one commonality might be that most women in that situation believe that it is too difficult to leave, that somehow they are at fault, and perhaps that life could be even worse if they left.

Your thinking might be similar in some ways, though this isn't easy to hear or acknowledge. Do you think it is too difficult to leave, that it is somehow your own fault that you cannot manage the stress, that life might be even worse if you were to take a different path?

The meaning translates into reasons why we can't. As I said, this meaning is very powerful and compelling; these reasons present themselves to us as the truth when they are not.

This is a point I would love to explore with you in much more detail. This is where the rubber hits the road, as you begin to explore your limiting beliefs and acknowledge the power they hold over everything you do and have in your life.

But if things had no meaning, well, what would that mean? How could we rely on anything anymore?

Rather than believing our world would spiral out of control, perhaps it would mean that we no longer had to make everything fit into our belief system; it would bring with it more clarity and freedom, an easiness towards life that many of us have not experienced since childhood. It would mean new and exciting opportunities that we were not able to see before.

Yet for most of us the old saying rings true: "better the devil I know."

Many people fear change. The unknown can be terrifying. We fear loss. We fear lack. At least we know what we have right now.

I can relate. I have been there. For many years I was trapped in this cycle. I had many fears, including fears around my financial security. Perhaps this is one of your fears as well.

Fears Around Finances

Many professionals might feel as though they are trapped in a golden cage. Before I made my career change, my income was above average. It allowed me to afford all the little luxuries of life I came to value significantly. I could pay for the mortgage, the car, the children's hobbies, an annual vacation, and did not have to count pennies when grocery shopping. There was even some left to save towards my retirement.

When I was thinking of leaving my practice, the fear of not being able to pay my mortgage anymore was very real. I felt that my obligations were fixed and I had to continue to find the same income to afford the life we all had become accustomed to. There seemed no choice but to continue in the same fashion.

Many of my colleagues are in a very similar situation. Expensive mortgage, children at private school, car loan, living expenses, and a multitude of other expenses keeping them locked into their current life, chained to a post that no longer fulfills them, robbing them of life itself.

Who says that these obligations are fixed? Society? Us?

None of this is fixed. You could sell everything, take the kids out of private school, move to Bali and buy a beach hut selling ice cream. I know it is not very likely that you would do this, and—though part of me fancies the idea of it—neither will I. But this is to illustrate that there are options, changes you can make if you allow yourself to see them.

Perhaps you wonder where any decision to change will lead you, and another burning question arises.

What Else Can I Do?

You are a highly skilled person. The skills you have are transferable. Transferable to a different position within medicine, or transferable to a position outside of medicine. You could consider working in research, for medical defense organizations, or the World Health Organization. Perhaps working for the courts has always been of interest to you, or you might want to support colleagues who are struggling. There are a multitude of options out there.

Thinking there is nothing else you can do is selling yourself short. Of course there are other things you can do, you could even continue to do the same job but with different conditions.

What is comes down to is your priorities. What is more important to you? How do you want to spend your time now? Not in 20 or 30 years when you can finally retire. Remember, now is all we have. It comes back to identifying what it is that you want in the first place.

This is a huge decision, and following your intuition can be helpful. Looking for the little spark of excitement that tells you that you're heading in the right direction.

Is there anybody in the world doing something that makes you think: "Wow, I wish I could do what they're doing!" This feeling is what you're looking for. This feeling, this wish, means you are looking in the right place. Often this is followed by: "Oh well, I'll never be able to do that." Those are your limiting beliefs talking. Question that, as that voice is not reliable. The person you admire was not born doing what they are doing. A journey led them there. Your journey will also lead you somewhere, and the direction you take now will determine the destination. It is never too late.

Societal Pressures

Our society puts enormous pressure on us. From a very young age we are exposed to certain values and dogmas. These become the bedrock of what we believe the world to be like. What we perceive as successful, how a woman should behave, the rules of society, and everything that determines how we live, fall into that category.

The truth is that besides the laws of physics, everything else is made up by people just like us, even the law of the land. We can see this easily by looking back in time. We now see as barbaric many customs that were commonplace not that long ago. And future generations will look at what we do now and wonder at the same thing.

The simple recognition of this fact is powerful. Again, it allows us to look at these rules more objectively and decide for ourselves if they fit with our own model of life.

The unspoken rule that you're expected to stay in your medical partnership until retirement held true until not that long ago. It was assumed that there must be something wrong with anybody who chose to leave.

I wonder what unspoken rules you adhere to? It is certainly worthwhile to spend some time questioning the rules we so readily adhere to. Do they really serve our well-being? Or do they simple serve the status quo?

Workplace Pressure

Part of the pressure we feel and a big obstacle to change is the pressure we feel at work. Medical professionals tend to be people with a very high commitment. We want to help, we want to contribute, we want to ease suffering. We do not want to let our colleagues and patients down, even to our own detriment.

Let me ask you a different question altogether. Imagine a person just like you came to seek medical advice from you. They tell you about the strains and stresses they are exposed to daily, they tell you about their lack of time to cook, exercise, and look after themselves. They tell you of the strain on their relationships, both at work and at home. What would you advise them?

Would you suggest they carry on as they are? For how long would you suggest they carry on? What would need to happen before you suggested they make a change?

Why do you think you should treat yourself differently from how you would treat one of your patients?

Putting ourselves first does not come easy, but it must be the starting point of any lasting change. This is not selfish, it is a necessity.

Identity

One of the biggest hurdles to creating change can be around identity. Who are you really? And who would you be if you changed your role or moved out of the profession altogether?

As a group of professionals, we tend to identify very strongly with being doctors. With this label comes certain assumptions, privileges, and status. We are an important part of our society, we make a real contribution to people—this role can be our main identity. The thought of changing or even leaving behind this identity can be scary, and for many doctors, an obstacle preventing them from making the right decision for them.

Who then are you, really?

Being a doctor is just a mask we wear. Your identity comes partially through your work, yes. But also through your relationships. Through your sexuality. Through your religion. Your political orientation. Your hobby. Your role as mother or father, son or daughter, caregiver. Whatever it might be.

These are roles we play, identities we take on for some time. But ask yourself who or what is beneath all of that. Allowing these roles to drop away, one by one, will bring you closer to your core, your true essence, or self, which is by nature spiritual.

Of course, we need to be able to take on these identities to fulfill our roles in society. There is nothing wrong with that, as long as we are aware that they don't completely define us.

Can't Appear Weak or Unknowing

This was one of my biggest obstacles. I had this acute sense that I always had to cope and be able to deal with every problem. The mere thought of not knowing something would strike panic in my heart.

There are many reasons for this, some personal and some professional. We all realize that is not possible to know everything. The key is to be aware of any gap in knowledge and address it appropriately. Yet for many doctors, the pressure of having to know everything is very strong. Not knowing can mean a loss of competence, a loss of respect, a loss of connection. It can lead to not asking the relevant and important questions, it can lead to isolation and increased fear. And it can just make your working day unpleasant.

As with most things, honesty is the best policy. Honesty with colleagues, with patients, and most importantly with yourself. We are human, we would not expect anyone else to be perfect, to know everything, but we often expect it from ourselves. Self-compassion is crucial in this context.

Perhaps you do not suffer from this affliction. I realized perfectly well that it's not possible to know everything, but somehow this did not stop me from feeling this pressure.

Internal vs. External Validation

For me it came down to seeking approval from others. In my work, I still associated the father I had never had with authority figures and trying to please them. All this to receive love and support, to feel I was cherished, wanted, and important.

Now I realize that validation needs to come from within. There will always be some people who love and admire what you do and others who feel the opposite. You cannot possibly please them all or try to make it right for everyone.

The validation you're seeking, the knowledge that it is ok to make a change, to live life according to your personal values and beliefs, needs to come from within.

It is here you will find all the strength, courage, and inspiration you need.

Key Points to Take Away

In this chapter, we discussed what might possibly hold you back from making the changes you desire.

We explored the meaning we give to everything that happens in our lives and realized that meaning and event are separate, that we can choose what meaning we attribute to these events. We spoke about fears that can hold us back and the importance of our identity.

One of the most important points right at the very end of the chapter was the call to seek validation from within. This will create the space and freedom you need to decide what is right for you and your life.

There is no doubt that you will encounter resistance on this journey. This is what we will explore in the next chapter.

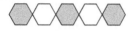

Chapter 5

Pushing Through Resistance

When I embarked on this journey to completely reinvent my life, to change what I do, to be empowered to make the choices that were right for me, I never truly believed I would get there. It felt incredibly scary, at times impossible, and the universe threw various obstacles in my way. These obstacles allowed me to get in touch with a deeper part of myself, with my limiting beliefs. I realized that what I saw around me was just the reflection of those beliefs. Only through the process of looking deeply was I able to let go of these beliefs and step into a new life.

"What you think—you become
What you feel—you attract
What you imagine—you create."
Buddha

This is one of my favorite quotes. There is so much wisdom and truth in this simple statement. It illustrates the power we all have, yet so often ignore or use wrongly. I'm not suggesting that we use it wrongly with conscious awareness. We simply have no real understanding or knowledge of the laws of the universe.

This universe is governed by very exact laws. Laws that allowed scientists to calculate the exact minute Apollo 11 would land on the moon. Though our knowledge of these laws is increasing all the time, there is still much we do not yet understand.

Not knowing or understanding them does not make these laws untrue though—they still apply and play out perfectly.

Let me give you Newton's second law of motion as an example. It states that the acceleration of an object is directly proportional to the magnitude of the net force in the same direction and inversely proportional to its mass. We also know that once an object is traveling with a certain velocity in a certain direction, it can be difficult to stop or change it.

We are in a similar situation as we seek to change the direction of travel our life is taking. The more we have invested, the faster we travel, the more difficult it will be to bring about change. Of course, there can be abrupt occurrences—such as illness or an accident—that bring about a sudden unexpected change, but this is not something we are looking for.

The aim of this book is to allow you to make conscious choices leading you to a life of choice, freedom, and happiness in a way that feels safe and manageable.

This process can feel uncomfortable. It is the resistance that seeks to keep you where you are. It is not change itself that is painful, but the resistance to change. But just because it feels scary and difficult does not mean it cannot be done.

Ability to Feel Uncomfortable

Many people see themselves as victims. They might not even be aware that this is what they are doing, but if you think that life is happening *to* you, then you have a victim mentality. This mentality does not make it easy for you to take charge of your life, as there won't be much you can do about it anyway.

There will come a time when this mentality will no longer serve you, and perhaps this is the place you are right now. The time has come to take charge of your life, to consciously create a life in alignment with your values and your purpose. Just be aware that this process can feel uncomfortable.

Being able to feel uncomfortable is a great skill when applied correctly. This feeling is different from the pain you feel as you carry on with a life no longer suited to you. This feeling heralds change; yet not knowing how this change can be made and exactly where it will lead can leave you feeling uncomfortable. It can have the power to derail the process should you allow this.

EXERCISE:
BEING THE OBSERVER

This is a great exercise you can use to help you with this uncomfortable feeling. It is our mind's job to move us away from pain and towards pleasure, so it comes quite naturally to want to shy away from these feelings. What is more powerful, though, is to simply observe the feeling and to understand more about it, without judging it or giving it meaning.

The exercise is simple. Find a quiet time and place to make yourself comfortable. Sit with your eyes closed and take a few deep breaths in and out. Allow yourself to relax more and more with every breath you take, with the rise and fall of your abdomen. As you relax more and more, imagine that you are going to the movies. See yourself walking into the theater. It's empty, you are the only guest. Take a seat of your choice and make yourself comfortable. On the screen, you will see your thoughts and feelings displayed. Just observe them as thoughts come and go, as feelings come and go. Do not judge, do not hinder them in any way, just observe. You might find that there are images you can see clearly, perhaps scenes that play out repeatedly. Perhaps you do not see anything, but only sense your feelings; you might have a sense of simply knowing. There is no right or wrong here, you cannot get it wrong if you simply observe the activity of your mind and allow thoughts and feelings to surface without any attachment to them.

Allowing, Surrender, Silence

As you do this exercise, you will realize that your thoughts and feelings come and go, but do not define you. There is a deeper, more central part of you that can observe what is going on without attachment.

Allowing this process is powerful. Eventually you will find that your mind will begin to quiet down. There will be fewer thoughts and fewer feelings which spring up on the screen of your mind.

In this place of allowing, surrender, and silence is immense power.

This exercise allows you to do two things. Firstly, it allows you to become truly aware of the fact that your thoughts and feelings are fleeting. They come and they go, they only have the power you give to them, only the meaning you allocate. In themselves they mean nothing, they are simply the activity of your mind, triggered by events, memories, and other thoughts.

Secondly, this exercise connects you with a deeper part of yourself. Being aware and rooted in this deeper aspect allows you to be much more grounded. It is as though you are at the bottom of the sea, in stillness and serenity, less buffeted by the changing winds and storms on the surface.

Connecting to this part will allow you to push through the resistance with much more ease and grace. You will be able to feel this uncomfortable feeling and understand that it only signals the changes to come, nothing more, and nothing less.

Trust

Connected to this deeper aspect of yourself, you will find that trust will be more available to you. Trust that your feelings of overwhelm do not mean there is something wrong with you, trust that your values and intuition will take you where you need to go. It is not your job to identify how you are going to get there, but only what it is that you will find in this place. This requires trust and surrender.

These were skills I had to fight for. I believe that most doctors don't find it easy to allow and trust in this way. In many ways, it goes against our training. It goes against evidence-based medicine, where you need clear and scientific evidence of a thing before it is given value or a voice.

Even the way I phrased it just now is a demonstration of this. I said I had to "fight for it." In truth, there is nothing to fight for. This is a process of allowing and surrender, a process of letting go of outdated beliefs and allowing yourself to connect again with this deeper part of you. It seems strange that I find it so much harder to let go of old stuff, rather than adding new stuff in. I wonder how this process is for you?

What Makes You Happy?
What Makes You Unhappy?

We have already identified what you want and how you want to feel. I would like to look more deeply at these things now.

Let us look specifically at what makes you feel happy and what makes you feel unhappy. Take a piece of paper and make a list of all the things you can think of that fit these descriptions in two columns. They can be big or small, personal or involving others.

What makes you most happy? What is it that you are really looking forward to? What fills your heart with joy?

Where exactly are the sources of your perpetual pain? Is it the work itself? Is it a specific colleague? Is it the workload? Something completely unrelated? Bring awareness to this—through this awareness, change is possible.

I believe it is our emotional life that reflects our success as human beings. We all aim for a happy and fulfilling life, and bringing consciousness to the exact things that influence this is crucial. Simply put, do more of what makes you happy and you will be happier. Do less of what makes you unhappy and you will be happier. You can begin to move in that direction immediately, since it does not necessarily require drastic changes.

For instance, maybe having dinner with your family makes you happy. Having brought awareness to this, you can plan to do it more often. How about having a family dinner every week? Or if spending time with your partner brings you joy, then have a fixed evening every week you can spend together. These things require planning and determination. They can be derailed easily. You might struggle with childcare or chores. There are a multitude of obstacles that can get in the way. Ultimately though, this is where you will find joy and happiness. Knowing what makes you happy and doing it; setting priorities and making them a reality.

The same is true for things that make you unhappy. Identify exactly what they are and then see how best to change them or remove them from your life.

Why is Change So Difficult?

It all sounds so easy, doesn't it? Alas, it's not, and there are very specific physiological reasons for this.

True change requires establishing new neural networks in the brain. These networks are created by thinking new and different thoughts and establishing different beliefs, feelings, habits, and behaviors. Through learning new information, we increase the synaptic connections in our brain. These new connections allow us to jump out of the current system or program. With these new connections, the brain can change, and with that our mind can also change. Learning is a quantum function of the mind, which makes it different from a computer system, which cannot do this. This is exactly what is happening as you read through this book.

However, simply learning new information or skills is not enough to make real change. Without reflection, contemplation, or action, these new neural connections are lost within days. The only way to really embed these new connections is to act on them, speak about the new learning, and demonstrate it until it can replace the old patterns.

One example here could be gratitude practice. Spending 10–15 minutes every day writing down 10 things you are grateful for will have immense benefits for your overall mood and state of mind. But the results will not be immediate.

Reaping benefits from a new practice takes time. The latest research from University College London suggests this process takes a total of 66 days. At least a third of those 66 days of doing something new will be difficult. Reading the book alone is not enough: you need to act on it, to make it your own.

Creating new neural connections requires a significant amount of energy. As survival has always been the number one priority of our mind, energy preservation is crucial.

This simple biological fact is one of the main reasons why change is so difficult. The body tries to preserve energy and therefore tends to fall back on automated processes which have already been established in the subconscious mind, even if these processes are not in our best interest. Included here are bad habits, such as overeating as a reaction to stress, lack of exercise, negative thoughts, and feelings of being overwhelmed and stuck. Many of these are automated and repetitive, simply recreated out of habit.

Having someone to hold you accountable can greatly speed up the process of creating positive and empowering habits, thoughts, and emotions. Having someone to hold the space for you as you move into your new life, a life of joy and ease, is of immense benefit. It is not strictly necessary though, and there are lots of things you can do yourself.

The Importance of Repetition

To overcome the body's and the mind's resistance, repetition is essential. Any behavior, habit, thought, or emotion you wish to have more of in your life needs to be repeated again and again. Even if it seems impossible that you will make it into a habit.

But you will, with baby steps. And baby steps are ok, as it is consistency rather than intensity which will win out in the end. One drop of water at a time, one step at a time, is all that is required. Eventually the new thoughts and emotions become automatic, leading to new actions and experiences. These in turn will become an unconscious skill or habit in the same way that driving a car became an automatic skill.

Your thinking and feeling are very important in this process. With every thought and emotion we are all adding to ourselves. In truth, we are each but a collection of information and energy, bound and expressed in matter. We are a part of the expansive universe and therefore our nature is also expansive.

Nonetheless, the biology of change can make the process quite hard. The simple need for energy preservation can throw up a huge amount of resistance. Suddenly all manner of reasons to stay as we are can come into our minds. It feels easier, safer, and so much more familiar. There is the illusion of certainty and safety. We might say to ourselves, "I can never change," "Who am I to be able to do this?" or something as simple as, "I do not have enough time," or "Things are fine as they are."

Firstly, notice that these statements are but beliefs; they are not the truth.

The best way to deal with these thoughts and emotions is to simply observe them, without attaching any meaning to them. Remember they only have the meaning you give to them. If left alone, these thoughts and emotions will come and they will go.

Choice

You always have the ability to choose, whether you know it or not. The beliefs that we hold determine the choices we make. Beliefs such as, "If I leave my job, I will not have enough money to pay for the mortgage." This may or may not be true, but we stay in our job regardless.

Independent of such big decisions, you can choose new thoughts, which will lead to new emotions, and in turn to new experiences.

Mentally rehearsing who we want to be creates the neurological changes in the brain. The unconscious mind cannot differentiate between these new thoughts we have about ourselves and what we believe actual reality to be. To the unconscious mind, everything within the mind is real. This is the reason we get really scared watching horror films: Your conscious mind knows it is just a film, but it feels real to your unconscious mind, giving you the thrill of the adrenaline rush as your body reacts to the images on the screen. In other words, by mentally rehearsing who we want to be we are priming our brain, making it much more likely to experience what we wish for ourselves.

An example of creating these new neural pathways is seeking pleasure in little things. Deliberately finding pleasure in having a hot shower, the first tea or coffee of the day, seeing the face of a loved one, being in nature are just a few examples of being consciously aware of enjoying what you are doing in the now. If you consciously seek pleasure in these simple things, you are training your brain to experience that pleasure, making it much more likely for the same experience to occur in unexpected ways.

The same is true if we are doing the opposite. The more complaining we do, the more anxiety we feel, the more sorry we feel for ourselves, the more likely that we'll feel that way in the future.

Functional MRI scanning of the brain shows no difference in brain activity whether an event is imagined or real. Your brain changes by thinking differently, and then both brain and body look as though the event has already occurred.

Athletes know this all too well. Mental training, rehearsing the moment of victory, plays a big role in their daily routine. Research has shown that athletes who do this mental practice have better performance outcomes.

Imagination is therefore one of the most powerful tools we have at our disposal, for better or worse. It is never "just" your imagination. What we imagine, we create.

The Flow State

There is a specific mental state called the flow state. Being in this state will propel you towards your goals quickly and seemingly effortlessly. It is defined as being fully immersed in what you are doing, having a feeling of energized focus in the process of this activity. It is a state of supreme creativity and joy.

"So how do I get into this state?" I hear you ask.

Much has been written and said about the flow state. Personally, I relate to how Vishen Lakhiani, Founder of

Mindvalley, describes it. He says that this state is the balance of two things: being happy in the now, and having a vision for the future.

Let's look at this in more detail, as it's very important. There are four states of mind which determine whether you are happy in the now or not and whether you have a vision for the future or not.

There are many people who have neither. They are not happy in the now, and they also have no inspiring vision for the future. I am sure you see many of these people in your consulting room. I certainly have. And there were certain parts of my life when I found myself in this same space. If you have never been there, let me tell you that it is the most uncomfortable and painful place you can find yourself in. It's a dark place. Depression lives here. Suicidal ideation lives here. Here, there is no point to life, and it can be the hardest place to leave.

Some people are happy with their life, but have no vision for where they would like to go, what they would like to achieve. This is a place where you can find yourself happy, yet unfulfilled. This is the current reality trap.

I strongly believe that human beings have the evolutionary need to grow and evolve. In this current reality trap, this fundamental human need is not addressed, and this will lead to an unfulfilled life.

The third possible state is when people have a great vision for the future, they can see and taste it already, and at the same time they are deeply unhappy with what they have right now. They are incredibly driven and purposeful, but also stressed and anxious in their daily life. As they reach one goal or milestone, another pops up immediately, and they find themselves chasing this elusive feeling of happiness and achievement forever. The aim here is to dissociate happiness from the vision. In other words, you are not depending on the achievement of your vision or goal for your happiness. You need to be happy *before* achieving your goal; happy while chasing your dreams. If you can do this, it leads you to the last state.

This is the flow state. Here you are happy right now, and at the same time have a great vision for your future. Happiness becomes a part of your journey, you can have great and inspiring goals, but do not depend on achieving them for your happiness.

Motivation

Motivation is important when moving towards any goal. Motivation is what you need when you don't feel like doing something. Motivation can give you the push you need to get going, but usually a significant amount of energy needs to be exerted to get any traction.

Yet there is something much better than motivation: inspiration and being in the flow state. It is in this state that your future reaches out to you and pulls you forward. There is no push required, no huge expense of energy to get started and to keep going. Here we have the mental state where you are being pulled into your future by the goals you have, and also being perfectly happy where you are right now. Strangely, it does not matter quite so much whether you achieve the exact goal you set out for yourself. The joy and happiness of the journey become much more important. You can adapt and expand your goals as you move towards them, but you are not dependent on achieving them for your happiness.

It is my belief that this is how life should be. It is this state which is natural for us. Unfortunately, our society does not allow this easily—for many reasons that go beyond the scope of this book. Nonetheless, you can endeavor to empower yourself, to find a way into this state and be there as much as you can. Like any skill, it does get easier with practice.

Achieving a State of Flow

There are many ways you can achieve a state of flow. Remember back to a time when you felt excited and happy in the now, and at the same time were looking forward to an exciting future. Perhaps as a student? Spending time at college with your friends, having a fun time, and studying for an exciting career ahead. I am sure there are many examples in your life. Remember how those moments felt. Make this feeling as real as you possibly can. Close your eyes and feel it, feel it in every cell of your body. Feel the joy and excitement, the zest for life. This is the feeling you are looking for.

Gratitude

There are many ways you can foster this flow state, and one of the most powerful ways is the expression of gratitude.

Regardless of how tough and exhausting your life can be, there will always be things to be truly grateful for. A warm bed to sleep in at night, heartfelt thanks from a patient, a walk in nature, the smile of a loved one, or having a loving pet are just a few examples. Expressing gratitude daily is associated with an increase in wellbeing and happiness, possibly even outperforming the effects of antidepressants. Gratitude anchors the good things into your life, causing you to have more energy, higher emotional intelligence, less depression, better sleep, and more social connection.

There are other effective ways to achieve and maintain the flow state, to change the emotional and energetic landscape of your being. Forgiveness and self-compassion deal with any issues arising from the past, whereas creative visualization and future dreaming help create a future aligned with your highest desires and values.

These are powerful techniques, and should I ever have the privilege to work directly with you, we can explore those in much greater detail.

Key Points to Take Away

I know how tough it can be to walk the path you have chosen to tread. I know how scary and seemingly impossible it can appear. I also know that you can achieve your goals despite these feelings.

You have explored in some detail what makes you happy and unhappy, and you realize that thoughts and feelings are fleeting and don't mean all that much, even though they sometimes don't seem that way. You have connected to a deeper part of yourself, where you find strength and power.

Perhaps most importantly, you understand the importance of being in a state of flow, to be happy in the now while having a vision for your future. Gratitude can be a powerful aid to you as you move forward on this journey. These tools will be helpful, but ultimately it is you and only you who can take each and every step into this future. Let's explore this further in the next chapter.

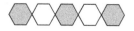

Chapter 6

Accountability

A few years ago, the following occurred on a regular basis. This is an account of a typical morning for me:

As I was about to open my eyes, I knew it was yet again very early in the morning, even though the early morning light shining though the gaps in the blinds might have deceived me.

Yep, it was 5 a.m. I was awoken by pressure. I couldn't even say where the pressure was, or why it was there. I was not in physical pain, but the pressure was certainly causing me discomfort, which you could call pain. Perhaps emotional pain, or mental pain. Perhaps even spiritual pain. I thought of the day ahead, the uncertainty around my work load; would I manage the complexity? What if I made a mistake, missed something? I just wanted to do something that would inspire me, not make me feel pressured and fearful.

What was I to do about this pressure? All I wanted was for it to go away, but it did no such thing. I felt vulnerable. I felt as though all my plans and ambitions were far out of reach. The old doubt was always near: "Who are you to make this big change?" I felt I couldn't stay where I was, yet did not want to move where I needed to go.

I acknowledged the pressure. I believed it was there to draw my attention to something. Something I needed to know, to realize, to heal, to let go of. Regardless of what I would find, I would not give up on my dream, my vision for me and my future.

As I pondered, I began to realize that my conflict was around wanting to please others, yet also go my own way. As I considered pursuing a life of my own choice, these old beliefs were coming up to the surface. The need to belong, the fear of not being able to survive, are some of the most powerful driving forces in our lives.

Mornings like this are now rare, but until not long ago, I would experience this on a regular basis.

It is the easiest thing to look to the outside world for reasons why our life is the way it is. There are so many different obvious reasons, and it seems to be just the way it is.

Yet, as I grappled with the responsibility for my own life, I realized that I was both the cause and the potential answer.

Responsibility

My fears, my limiting beliefs, and the subsequent feelings of discomfort, pressure, and pain were all created by me. No one else. That was a tough realization for me to wrap my head around. Yes, my life experiences and especially my childhood had instilled certain beliefs in me, and when I thought of these beliefs they made perfect sense to me. But now I realized that they were all based on subjective interpretation of events, not the truth. I was no longer a child, it was now up to me to look at my beliefs, my life, my ambitions, and decide where I wanted to go and who I would choose to be.

There is this saying: "With great power comes great responsibility." I have always felt this should be the other way around: "With great responsibility comes great power."

Think about it: As soon as you take responsibility for something, you have also placed yourself in a position to do something about it. You can no longer be a victim. If you give the power to outside circumstance, then it's up to outside circumstance to determine where you are headed. Obviously, no one has total control over all events in their world. But you have a lot more power over your own choices, your own thoughts and emotions than you might allow or admit.

As soon as you decide it is you who holds the responsibility, it also becomes you who can do something about it. With this comes the risk of failure—and you wouldn't have anyone else to blame for that failure. But then, it's also you who suddenly has the risk of succeeding.

Of course, our childhoods have a huge influence over everything we believe and experience. But once we are adults, the responsibility for our lives falls to us.

Let me remind you that responsibility does not equal fault. Taking responsibility does not mean you should feel blame, shame, or guilt.

If we take full responsibility for all our thoughts, emotions and actions, from a place of self-compassion, we place ourselves into a position of choice. This opens doors to us we might never have known are there.

The Power of Thinking

Our thoughts are more powerful than we admit to ourselves. Thoughts become things. Everything starts with a thought. All great inventions once lived purely in the minds of their creators before you could find any physical evidence of their existence. Sanitation, the moon landing, and the Internet, to give just a few examples.

The same was true for my thoughts of creating a different life for myself, away from the stresses and strains of working flat out in a system that was damaging to me and my patients. The same is also true of your thoughts about creating a life full of choice and ease. It is not yet in physical existence, but your thoughts bring you closer to your goal.

Thoughts are things. Thoughts are real.

What we continuously think about can become physical reality. This is a process that takes time and focus. One of the reasons we are not aware of the creative power of our thoughts is this time lag. By the time something we have thought about a lot comes into being, we have lost the connection between the thought and its manifestation. Or else we simply do not focus on and pursue a thought frequently enough for it to manifest physically.

This is like going to the travel agent, but being unable to decide on a vacation destination. First you decide on Italy, then Egypt, then California. In the end you will stay at home, because the travel agent is unable to book the trip for you due to your indecision and lack of focus.

The same might also be true about your thoughts about your future. I know, because this was true for me. For a very long time I thought about what I wanted to change in my life, but I also wanted to stay where I was. In other words, my thoughts were not consistent.

Little Acts of Creation

Let me impress upon you a very important fact: Thoughts are created. The creator of your thoughts is you. This places the power to create and to change right into your own hands.

We are creative beings by nature. We truly create our experience of the world. The more you think similar thoughts, the stronger the thought forms become, and the likelier it is that it will manifest into your life. This is particularly the case if emotion is used to power these thoughts.

Let me repeat an important point, which we spoke about in the last chapter. A thought is a word-based frame. Thinking the same thoughts activates the same memory circuit in the brain, and if done repeatedly, we begin to think it is the truth. This is because it becomes a pattern, hardwired into the neural circuit of the brain. The stronger the pattern becomes, the less likely it is that alternative neurons or circuits will be activated.

When we think a certain thought often enough, it seems that there is nothing else and therefore it must be the truth. You are already doing this. We are all doing this with every thought we think. The question here is whether your thoughts support you in your vision, or hinder you.

The Power to Choose Better Thoughts

Change will be much easier as the need to cling to what we think is true diminishes. The need to be right, as well as the need to convince others of our truth, also diminishes, as we begin to appreciate that everyone's truth is real to them.

We each have 40–60,000 thoughts every single day, and up to 90% of these thoughts are the same thoughts we had yesterday. Thinking these same thoughts continues to strengthen the same circuit, making it more likely that the thoughts are being repeated. It is believed that up to 80% of most people's thoughts are negative in nature. This is a staggering and bewildering percentage.

Negative thoughts have been shown to activate the fear center, the amygdala we spoke of in a previous chapter. These negative thoughts shut down our motivation and awareness centers. The stress response can be triggered by thoughts and beliefs, even those we are not aware of.

We all have negative thoughts. That is normal. The aim is not to eliminate them completely. The aim is to increase our awareness of them.

With awareness and the right tools comes a choice. The choice is whether you continue with your current thinking or change it, thus creating a different outcome, a different experience. A healthy mind can go back and forth between negative and positive thoughts and then come to an evaluation, and eventually to a decision, around the object of these thoughts.

Mostly thoughts of worry, fear, and doubt are based on memories from the past, either real or imagined. This is how we keep recreating the same or similar circumstances again and again.

The future is not yet here. There is nothing to say that it must be based on the past, unless we take our memories from the past and project them into the future. This is done by thinking the same thoughts repeatedly, thus creating the same outcome. But we don't have to follow that path.

Beliefs

As we have already heard, the issue with repeatedly thinking the same thoughts is that they become beliefs.

A belief is something we hold to be true about us or the world around us. Very often we see a belief as a fact, even though, in most instances, it's not. Beliefs can be formed in accordance with our thinking or with reality as we see it.

Beliefs can be taught or established through our imagination. Beliefs are formed as we give meaning to what is happening to and around us. This meaning is then powerfully reinforced as we continue to interpret our experiences through the lens of our beliefs. In other words, it is our beliefs that shape our experience.

Collective beliefs are often seen as facts. But simply because many people believe something to be true does not make it so. An obvious example was the common belief that the earth is flat, or at the center of the universe. Perhaps there are certain common beliefs you might have whose validity it might be worthwhile to question. The belief that you cannot make a change is just that, a belief. It is not the truth.

Beliefs shape our world to a much greater extent than most of us will admit. The reason for this is that we tend to act in accordance with our beliefs. This is a very crucial point for you to understand. It is like a pivot, which has the power to completely change your life and your future.

We act in accordance with our beliefs. This means that we seek in the world anything which will confirm the truth of what we believe. The world reflects the sum of the beliefs we hold. Our mind will automatically hone in on the events and nuances that strengthen and validate what we thought in the first place. This happens unconsciously and at lightning speed.

If our belief system is self-critical, then we notice the frown more than the smile. We also pay more attention to the complaint rather than the comments of appreciation.

Beliefs can either be empowering or self-limiting. Let me give you some examples of both.

Empowering beliefs: I am good enough. I am capable. I can cope with what life throws at me. I am lovable. The world is a friendly place. I can live a fulfilling life moving towards my goals. I can have a career giving me joy and happiness.

Disempowering beliefs: I am unworthy. I am not good enough. The world is a nasty and dangerous place. I will never amount to anything. No one will love me for who I am. Things will never change for the better. It is impossible.

If you really look at them, all these beliefs are subjective. Not only are these negative beliefs subjective, they are also generalizations. Notice the "never" or "always" that you might use in the expression of your beliefs.

Unconscious Beliefs

We all hold a large quantity of unconscious beliefs—beliefs we are not aware of. Quite a few of the beliefs I have listed earlier might be unconscious. Some unconscious beliefs are very common and many people hold them.

Among the most common are "I am not worthy," "No one truly wants me," and, "If I try I am going to fail," as well as "Making mistakes is bad."

Even though these beliefs are unconscious, your life will mirror those you have right back to you. The language you use when describing yourself or the world is one way to see these unconscious beliefs.

The Importance of Language

The language we use is an indicator pointing to the underlying beliefs we hold. This is the reason why it is so crucial to listen to what you say to yourself; to listen to this inner voice, to become the observer. As you become aware of your beliefs, you can review and alter them.

Beliefs are like the walls of a house. They form the structure and limitations of everything you experience in life. The walls of your belief system can restrain, limit, confine, and restrict. Or they can set you free. If you don't like your current living arrangements, so to speak, you always have the option to rebuild by dismantling old and outdated beliefs and replacing them with new and empowering ones.

No one will give you permission to do this. You cannot wait for permission to be given by others, you need to give it to yourself. This is your life we are talking about, no one else's. Only you can make the changes you are seeking, only you have the power.

Undermine or Empower

The words you say to yourself are the most powerful you will ever hear. Often this dialogue happens in the back of our minds, without much conscious awareness. These are the internalized voices of our parents and care-givers, the school friends or bullies we encountered, teachers, and all other influential people.

Listen to yourself. Are you kind to yourself, or critical? Compassionate or commandeering? If you spoke to your best friend the way you speak to yourself, would she like to remain your best friend?

Harsh, hurtful, critical words you tell yourself repeatedly are a major cause of low mood, anxiety, and depression. Self-praise, on the other hand, is incredibly powerful as there is no underlying agenda; it can massively increase your self-esteem.

Some scientists argue that verbal suggestions influence us on a cellular level. It is the cell membrane that acts as the brain of the cell, controlling which part of the genome is expressed. The environment, both internal and external, has a huge influence on the cell membrane, and as such it is possible that even thoughts can influence how our genome is expressed. It has also been suggested that our brain makes up 80% of what we perceive as our environment, and that we spend a large portion of the day in a trance state to allow this environment-building to happen.

Our minds respond to the words and images we create in our heads, and this process is very much within our control. It might feel unfamiliar or strange, but that does not mean it cannot be done.

Self-Talk

Choose empowering self-talk rather than indulging in feeling sorry for yourself or belittling yourself.

I can give you a list of the words and phrases I spoke on a regular basis while still in the middle of my stressful job. This list is in no particular order: "This is hell, stressed, not coping, knackered, done in, exhausted, overwhelmed, it's too hard, agony, nightmare, pushing me to the limit, it's going to kill me, disaster, driving me insane, too hard," and so on. Any of this sound familiar?

The language we use determines the way we see our reality. I can tell you that using these words certainly did not improve how I felt. Until you can change your working life to suit you better, use better language to cope with your current reality. Say, "I have chosen to do this and I have chosen to feel great about it." Say, "I am enough," "I can cope," and, "I have the power to change."

"I am"

These two little words are perhaps the most important of them all. As A. L. Kitselman said:

"The words "I am" are potent words. Be careful what you hitch to them.

The thing that you are claiming has a way of reaching back and claiming you."

Changing the language you use is essential as you move towards your ideal life, a life filled with joy and ease. The language you use is but the expression and mirror of your state of being. If you change one, you automatically change the other. You will begin to realize that you are the creator of your life, not at the mercy of circumstance.

The Questions We Ask Ourselves

Have you noticed that the questions you ask yourself are mostly answered? Just spend a moment to think what sort of questions you are asking yourself on a regular basis. I can tell you what sort of questions I used to ask myself. "What did

I do to deserve this?" "Why is my life so full of stress and anxiety?" or, "Will this never end?"

The universe answered all my questions. I saw the reasons and justification for my suffering all around me. I understood why my life was so full of stress and anxiety. And I carried on for what seemed like forever.

Now the questions I ask myself are very different. Now I wonder what amazing experiences I will have today. Now I ask how I can best help my clients step into a life of freedom and choice. Now I ask which amazing surprise is just around the corner.

All your questions are answered. Make sure you ask the ones you truly want the answers to.

Daily Choices

This process is more than language and questions, though. It is language translated into beliefs, habits, and actions. Daily small choices are very important. It is those small daily choices that will ultimately paint the tapestry which is your life.

Are these small and daily choices consistent with your life vision?

I can give you a few simple examples. Eating a whole tub of ice cream is not consistent with the vision of being fit, slim, and strong. Never listening to your partner is not consistent with the vision of having a loving and trusting relationship. Carrying on with your current job without looking for alternatives is not consistent with the vision of having a self-determined, joyful future career.

I know you can do this. Do you want to know why I know this? Because I did it. Because I successfully faced these struggles, which seemed insurmountable. I am no different from you. If I can achieve it, so can you.

EXERCISE:

There is a simple yet powerful exercise you can do, which has the potential to make a real difference in your life in a short amount of time.

Every morning I want you to write down five small goals you want to achieve that day. If your mornings are hectic and stressful, do this last thing at night for the following day. It does not have to be anything huge; small goals will suffice. The important part is to commit to achieving them before you retire for the night.

Let me give you some examples. Part of this list could be one or two things that make you really happy, such as spending time with loved ones, having a massage or a walk in nature. Your goals could be around starting to investigate an alternative career, ways to reduce your hours, finding an alternative source of income. Or it could be around your health, diet and exercise.

If you stick to this daily list, you will have achieved a phenomenal amount within just a few weeks or months. Imagine keeping this up for years to come! Your life will not be recognizable.

Key Points to Take Away

We have explored the importance of taking responsibility for your own life. This includes the awareness that thoughts are things. Thoughts are created, and you are the creator of our own thoughts. Though possibly difficult at first, it is in your power to choose different thoughts, which will translate into different feelings and ultimately different actions, behavior and experiences.

The language you use every day is a powerful tool, and using this to your advantage will make a huge difference in your life. Asking empowering questions will bring different and new energy into your life, along with joy and excitement.

Certain steps are required to make your life vision a reality. I have already given you a powerful exercise, and we will dive deeper into this pursuit in the next chapter.

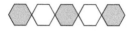

Chapter 7

Creating the Future

Now we will bring it all together. Everything you have learned about yourself, your goals, your vision, and your values. You understand why change can feel so difficult, but you are aware of the cost of not making this change. You have the tools and you understand where your possible obstacles lie. And you understand the most important piece of the puzzle—it is up to you and no one else to make this change. It is entirely in your power to create a life filled with joy; a life where your work supports you, rather than drains you.

I would be lying if I told you that my journey was easy. It certainly was not. There were many times when I thought of giving up, when it felt too hard and seemed impossible. Yet, here I am with a different life, much happier and more empowered, able to choose for myself how I spend my time. And the same thing happened for many of my clients.

It always starts with the simplest of things.

Deciding

Yes, this is what it took. Simply making the decision: deciding what I wanted, putting my stake down on the map, and then moving towards it. This decision was made in an instant, with conviction and clarity. You have explored the reasons why you want to do this. You know where the road will lead if you do not make a change. These reasons are the fuel which will propel you towards your goal. Keep them in mind, and look at the list you created in chapter three (the list of what you want and how you want to feel) every day.

Your choice could be to stay in your current practice, but reduce your hours or commitments. Your choice could be to go part-time in your current job and use the time you have freed up to build a different career or take on a different role that fills you with passion. Perhaps you choose to leave your post and move to a different area to start afresh. Perhaps you decide to leave medicine behind altogether and travel for a while, before embarking on something completely new and different.

Regardless of your choice, there will be a part of your mind that will want to convince you that it can't be done. It will be very convincing, and what this part of you says will make perfect sense. Yet, despite this, you know deep down that it's not true.

You don't need to worry about the how. What you want is so much more important than how you're going to get there.

So, make the decision. Do it right now. What do you really want? How committed are you to getting it?

I wrestled with my ego for a long time over this point. Every time I thought I had made this decision, it would say "Yes, but…." The "but" seemed so true. I argued with myself, looked at the issue with compassion, tried to have the better reason for doing it, but in the end, it was quite simple. I simply decided. Regardless of the counterarguments, the fear, the worry, and all the other reasons.

Commitment

Once you have made the decision, it's important to commit fully. Behave as if this new life was already reality. Speak as though the outcome you want is inevitable. Rejoice in the freedom, new experiences, and quality of life that is yours to claim. Right now!

I know you are committed as a person. You would not have gotten to where you are otherwise. You were committed to your studies, and now you are committed to your patients, colleagues, and job. This would be wonderful, if only your current circumstances, your job with all its obligations and pressures, were not this painful.

The time has come to think about yourself, to commit to your own well-being, your own happiness. The time has come to fill up your own cup until it overflows. And from this overflow you can give freely without depleting yourself. I know it's a very old analogy, but it holds true. You need to put on your own oxygen mask first. If you die, you can help no one.

Creative Visualization

Now that the decision has been made, it is important to be clear about what you want, to fill in the detail. What do you want to experience? How do you want to feel? What do you envision yourself doing in your new life? In what way do you want to contribute to the world?

This is the vision you have for your life. It will pull you into the future. Having a vision differentiates humanity from animals, who can only base their decisions and reactions on what is happening in the now.

Perhaps difficult conversations need to be had and other people will be disappointed by your choices. Having a vision allows you to overcome these obstacles. You know why you are doing what you are doing, and this makes all the difference.

Spend some time every day visualizing your perfect future as clearly as possible. Pretend it is already reality. Remember that the unconscious mind cannot differentiate between fantasy and reality. Use all your senses. What do you see? What are you doing? Make it colorful and bright. Are there any sounds you can hear? What do you sense, smell, or taste?

One of the most important aspects of your visualization is the emotional content. Emotion provides the energy, it is the fuel. It allows you to step into the flow state, this state of effortless creativity. Feel in the now how you will feel once it has all come into reality. The joy, freedom, and ease feel so beautiful. You can sense the pressure and stress leaving your body more and more with every deep breath you take. Do this right now. Simply close your eyes and spend five to ten minutes doing this.

Creative visualization is powerful. It is a well-known tool many people use to influence their reality and manifest their life vision. Connecting with your dream life on a regular basis brings it ever closer into physical reality.

Expectancy

To speed the process up significantly, it is helpful to develop a mental attitude of expectancy. Even though your outer reality is not yet what you want it to be, you must know without a doubt that it will be. You expect this to be the case, without any wavering, with absolute certainty.

When you go to a restaurant and order a drink, you know your drink will arrive. You expect this to be the case, even though there is no physical evidence of it just yet. When you order your dinner, again you know the waiter will bring it to your table. This is the feeling I want you to develop when it comes to your ideal future. Know what it will be and watch it unfold.

While it is important to have this expectancy, it is also important not to be fixed on how your vision will materialize. The restaurant analogy is helpful again in this context. Let's say you ordered lasagna. You know what you can expect, yet you would not dream of going into the kitchen and telling the chef how to cook it—you trust that she knows what she's doing. Going into the kitchen would no doubt throw a wrench in the works, and the same is true for your life vision. Know the *what* and leave the *how* for the universe to figure out. Trust.

Goal-Setting and Strategy

You have your vision. You know with certainty it will come into being. You have thought it through, you expect it, yet you allow it to unfold. You know what it feels like, and this is the perfect starting point. Without this starting point, you could not get there—but on its own it is not enough.

Creating your vision and having an attitude of expectancy is half the battle—the other half is making it happen. You need to move from designing your vision to building it as your reality. Your vision needs to be broken down into small, achievable steps that you can implement and make real one step at a time. These are goals we are talking about, not mere wishes or hopeful thinking. These could be the small daily goals you learned to set for yourself in the last chapter.

You will be very familiar with this process. Most likely it will form an essential part of keeping up to date with the knowledge within your specialty. Without chunking your overall vision down into small achievable pieces, it might seem too overwhelming, too difficult to accomplish. Remember that even the most amazing journey, the biggest adventure, starts with a single step.

Developing SMART goals will serve you well. Goals that are Specific, Measurable, Achievable, Realistic (as well as rewarding) and Time-bound. Take one action, even if it's the smallest thing, that moves you towards your goal every single day. If you can achieve five small goals every day, your progress will be much faster.

This is where most people and most plans fail. It all sounds great, and you can visualize and plan all day, but your new life will not miraculously plop into your lap.

What you are trying to achieve is the perfect balance of opposites. Being active and passive, doing and thinking, taking control and surrendering. All these are skills that are essential and need to be balanced in a beautiful dance, always moving, yet seemingly still. Experiment, try it out without taking it too seriously. You will learn every step of the way until you become masterful.

Ask yourself what you need to achieve your goal. Which habits do you need to develop? What attitude must you embody? Which exact steps do you need to take? Who can support you? Who can you ask for advice or help?

Then, one step at a time, your vision will come into being.

This is exciting! I feel so excited for you. We all have a need to exert control over our lives; self-determination is an important human need.

Brain Plasticity, Neurogenesis, and Change

There is no reason why this can't be done. When I went to college in the 1990s, we were taught that the brain is no longer able to change and grow once adulthood had been reached. It was thought that all synaptic connections were fixed, like set concrete.

Scientists and the medical community also believed that brain cells could not be replaced. If they died for whatever reason, it was an irreplaceable loss.

Neither of these assertions has turned out to be true. The brain and nervous system are truly incredible. No manmade computer could ever rival or equal the complexity and interplay of our nervous system. There are over 100 billion neurons within your brain. This high number allows for the incredible processing capability of the brain.

We now understand neurogenesis much better. Even though most of this takes place in the period before birth, it has been shown that even in adults, new nerve cells are born in multiple areas of the brain.

And then there is neuroplasticity. This is the brain's ability to form new connections throughout life, thus reorganizing itself. In other words, the brain is malleable. It does *not* set like concrete.

This is great news indeed. This means the brain can and does change. It means we have unlimited capacity to grow and change.

Change is not only possible, it is inevitable. The only question is whether you allow change, or direct it. I believe it is important to be able to both allow and direct. We tend to resist change. This is like resisting the fast-flowing current of water. Ultimately it's not possible, but will cost a huge amount of energy and cause pain and discomfort.

Resistance and the resulting pain are closely linked to a need to control. We feel if only we could control what is going on around us, life would be so much easier. In fact, the opposite is true. We can only control our own responses, our own thoughts and emotions. It is through this that the outer reality will begin to appear different to us. There is a subtle yet powerful difference between controlling and directing.

The Nature of Reality

What is real? What is reality?

Everything that is out there in the physical world is interpreted through our five senses. This allows our nervous system to create an image of what we perceive to be out there within our own mind. What we think of as the world is only our interpretation of the world.

Studies have shown that many more nerve cells are activated in the brain when we see, hear, or feel something than there are cells within the sensory systems alone. This means that our mind is interpreting what we see and referencing it to the existing memory bank. Not only this, but emotional centers are also activated. In other words, whatever we are exposed to, our mind looks for how we might have felt about similar experiences in the past and what this could mean for us in the present or future.

But what does all this mean?

It means that what we have within our mind is but an interpretation of what is out there, and it can never be objective or true in the absolute sense. Everything we experience is colored by our mind. Colored by our previous experiences, our thoughts, emotions, expectations, beliefs, hopes, and fears. Colored by the meaning we have given to past events as well as expected future events. Our eyes are not only a lens through which we see the world, they seem to also function as a projector. And this projection is different for every single human being on the planet. You are truly unique, no one else has the same experience of the world as you.

It also means that the world is but a mental construct, existing in your mind. I know it doesn't feel like that. It feels real. It's a powerful illusion and explains much of the world's conflicts, as most people are convinced that their interpretation of reality is the only possible one.

The Truth Behind Manifestation

Modern physics asserts that there is no matter, only energy. Quantum mechanics has the scientific proof for this. We know beyond doubt that the whole of the universe is made up of energy. We know that energy cannot be destroyed, but only transmuted. The universe can be likened to a giant mind of which we are a crucial part.

Quantum mechanics speaks of a particle *of* motion, which is energy, rather than a particle *in* motion, which would be matter. Eastern philosophies never had this concept of matter in the same way Western cultures did. Ancient yogis always maintained that the smallest particles of matter are, in fact, vortices of energy. And it is exactly this vortex of energy that creates the illusion of the material, the illusion of matter.

This means that we live in a non-material universe. Particles of matter are nothing but particles of pure movement, where nothing really exists that moves. Nothing material anyway: only energy. These particles are more like thoughts. They are not things. They can be likened to acts of consciousness and not material substance.

"Today there is a wide measure of agreement that the stream of knowledge is heading towards a non-mechanical reality; the Universe begins to look more like a great thought than a great machine."
Sir James Jeans

You might wonder why I am bringing this up at this point in the book. To many people with a scientific background this sounds like mumbo jumbo. Yet modern physics asserts these points. Though I do not fully understand all the experiments and arguments, I believe they are true.

What it means is that reality is much more fluid than we assume. It means that, if we change how we perceive the world, the world will change. It means we have much more power over our experience of the world than we ever thought. This is the reason I am raising this point now. I want you to understand that you truly can change your life.

Freedom and Quality of Life

It is up to you to claim this power as your own. The choice is yours. You can choose to allow circumstances to dictate your beliefs, thoughts, and emotions, or you can take charge of your life. By being fully responsible, you will greatly empower yourself. Who says you must stay in a system that is so destructive? Allow yourself to see other options, better choices, a life of self-determination.

The old paradigms will not let you go without a fight, though, I can promise you that. The voice in your head will argue that it cannot be done, that it is not true, that you need to remain as you are. After all, what you've done all these years has kept you alive. Making a big shift like this feels overwhelming and scary. Yet it can be done. It can be done with intention, repetition, and support.

The reward will be freedom. The freedom to choose how you want to live your life. The freedom to create a job or position that is fulfilling and manageable. The freedom to enjoy your life, rather than allow fear and worry to dictate a large part of it.

Ultimately, the quality of your life is what it is all about. Give yourself permission.

EXERCISE:
MEETING YOUR FUTURE SELF

I would like to finish this chapter with a powerful exercise. This exercise is best done when you are alone and unlikely to be disturbed, perhaps first thing in the morning or last thing at night before you go to bed.

Sit or lie down, and imagine that you are going to meet your future self. Your future self has achieved everything you are planning to achieve, perhaps five years into the future. A career which is fulfilling and manageable; in fact more than manageable, a career which fills you with joy as you look forward to work, rather than dread it. A home life that makes you happy and connected. Enough time to look after yourself in the perfect way for you. This might involve travel, spending time with friends and family, or taking up a new hobby.

Imagine your future self walking up to you, connecting with you. This is your opportunity to question your future self and ask how she has managed to make all the changes so successfully. Spend enough time with this exercise to make this experience as real as possible.

Should we ever work together, we can do this exercise together as a guided meditation. This is incredibly powerful and can have a real impact on how your future unfolds.

Key Points to Take Away

All the work from previous chapters has led you to deciding. In the end, it is as simple as that. Deciding to have a better life, deciding to make a change.

Though having the right thoughts and emotions and being aware of your values is important, it is equally important to realize that your new life needs to be created by you. Setting achievable goals and moving towards your life vision every single day will bring it into being. The perfect balance of allowing and creating means you're not insisting on your life vision manifesting in one way only. This allows you to enter a flow state and move with ease and joy towards the manifestation of your vision.

You now have all the pieces of the puzzle to creating and manifesting your vision. There is just one hurdle left, which we will discuss in the next chapter.

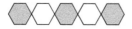

Chapter 8

The Last Hurdle

What is your next step going to be? How will you make your new life a reality? Are you ready to create your new life? Will you give yourself permission?

I hope so. It is yours for the taking.

To overcome the last hurdle, you need to believe it is possible. This is all that's required. Without doubt, without hesitation, simply knowing it to be true, and then taking steps in the right direction. This can be the hardest part. And sometimes we need help with this. We need someone to hold us accountable, to reflect what is really going on.

You know all you need to know. You feel and understand the truth of your situation. Yet there might still be a little part deep within holding you back.

When I was writing this book and making huge changes in my life, this was the situation I found myself in. It was not that I did not know how to do it—I had been studying personal development, the psychology of change and hypnotherapy for years; I was a trained hypno-psychotherapist and Rapid Transformational Therapist in addition to being a doctor. I understood painfully well why I needed to change my work commitments. I knew if I did nothing, my quality of life would continue to be severely affected both right now and in years to come. My health and my relationships were going to continue to suffer. Ultimately, I would not serve my patients in this way.

Yet part of me just could not believe it would be possible, part of me chose to stay stuck. I had to take a very hard look at myself and ask how this old pattern of behavior was serving me.

How Is Your Current Situation Serving You?

We can get stuck for several reasons. Sometimes we don't know how to make a change. I knew how to and you know this as well. Sometimes circumstances demand that we plan carefully and put an exact plan into motion. Sometimes though, what we do serves a deeper purpose, it is an unconscious choice. Though very painful, we choose to remain in the current situation.

This was the case for me. I chose to stay where I was, because I was afraid. I was afraid to fail, but I was even more afraid to succeed. If I was successful and my book and coaching program sold well, I would have to step up to the plate. I would risk not being good enough. I would risk rejection. No doubt some people would love my work and others would hate it. That's just life. I had to learn that this was not a reflection of me, but of the person making this judgment.

I had to learn that it's ok to seek validation from within, that I don't need external validation. I was making excuses for myself and being stuck served me well. Choosing to stay stuck allowed me to avoid looking at these deeper issues.

Eventually though, I reached a turning point. I had already made some significant changes in my life, but decided that I needed support to deal with these last deep-rooted issues. I hired a coach. It was not easy to face up to my issues. It was not easy to hear that I allowed my ego to run the show. To hear that staying stuck meant that I chose not to help you. That I put my own egotistic needs before truly stepping into my power to serve.

So, ask yourself, why are you still stuck? Why have you not already left this place? Why do you choose to remain? What are you afraid of?

Perhaps nothing, and you are powerfully stepping into your new life. This is my wish for you. My wish is that you take the new knowledge you have discovered about yourself and use it to create the life of your dreams. I know you can.

Perhaps though, like me, you would like some support and help on this journey.

If you have any specific questions about your personal situation or about any of the content of this book, I would be delighted to talk to you.

Simply email me: maritta.philp@gmail.com. You can also visit my website, which is www.marittaphilp.com, to complete a questionnaire giving you more clarity about your current situation. Once you truly understand your specific situation, your pain points, your dreams, and ambitions, you can figure out the best next steps, regardless of where they will lead you, with my help or without.

The Mind

We spoke a lot about the mind in this book. If you can truly understand how the mind works, you can instruct it and communicate with it to empower you on this path. When I trained as a Rapid Transformational Therapist, my teacher, Marisa Peer, taught us that there are three important aspects to consider.

We already discussed how the mind likes what is familiar. This alone is a powerful motivation not to change anything. Anything new is potentially dangerous or threatening. We have the fear that making the change will leave us worse off. The truth is that you can make anything familiar, by using the techniques we discussed in this book. Use your imagination, practice how you want to feel, and take time to enjoy the small things in life every single day.

Secondly, your mind also responds powerfully to the words and images you create. The stronger the image and associated emotion, the more powerfully your mind will react. So be aware of the language you use and the impact of the images you create. You can take control simply by increasing your awareness and making different choices.

Lastly, the mind does what it thinks you want it to do. It is important to give your mind very clear instructions to inform it of what you want. Remember the example of booking a vacation or choosing a meal in a restaurant. You will only get what you want if you can clearly articulate what that is. The first step of this communication must be with your own mind.

Who Holds the Power?

This is the big question. Who holds the power? Who have you given the power to? Whose life is it we're talking about?

Reclaim your power with compassion and kindness towards yourself and others.

Life is an amazing adventure. We only have one shot at this particular life. Though I believe it is never too late to make a change, I also know that time passes quickly. You will never get your time back. The time really is now.

Let me finish this chapter with a powerful and well-known saying.

"If you always do what you have always done,

you will always get what you have always gotten."

It is madness to think you can get a different outcome by doing the same thing. People often wonder why things are no different, yet fail to consider that they keep repeating what they have always been doing.

Step into your new life! With or without my help. I know you can.

Conclusion

What a journey we have been on. I am so thrilled that you trusted me to be your companion on this journey.

I hope you come away with new insights, deeper understanding, and hope. Hope that the life of your dreams is just around the corner. Hope that you can make it a reality.

No, more than just hope. Clarity. Knowledge. Certainty.

I know and trust that you can.

We have explored many different aspects of this process. Ultimately, all the power lies with you. If you understand that your life is the result of the small decisions you make every day, traveling on a course set by your beliefs and intentions, and colored in the now through your language, thoughts and emotions, I feel I have done my job well. Life is subjective. These things are much more under your control than you might ever have thought.

This also means there is no one else to blame. More accurately, there is no one to blame, full stop. Blame is never helpful. What is helpful is to achieve clarity about what you want and why you want it, and then go ahead and create what you want one step at a time.

What this change entails depends on you and your priorities. Perhaps patient care is as important to you now as it always was and you cannot see yourself in a non-clinical position. That is great. Your skills are very much in demand. You will be able to find a position that allows you to do what you love without damaging you beyond repair.

Perhaps you have decided to leave medicine. This is also a valid decision. You have the most amazing and transferable skills, and now is the time to dream big. I feel excited for you as you step into a new adventure.

You must understand though, that reading this book alone will not bring you the results you seek. The exercises are part of the process, as is your willingness to try new and different things. To step out of your comfort zone, to allow yourself to be stretched without feeling panic, to see new opportunities, to let go and surrender.

You need to understand that there will be resistance and there will be times when you want to give up, believing it is not so bad after all.

Believe me when I tell you that this can be overcome.

My Wish for You

My wish for you is that you immerse yourself fully into this life.

My wish for you is that you realize your own power to make the changes you seek.

My wish for you is that your life is filled with joy and happiness, a zest for life, and excitement as you envision and create a life reaching your fullest potential.

My thoughts are with you on this journey. May you travel well.

Acknowledgments

Writing this book has been an amazing journey of growth. It has been challenging in more ways than I can ever tell, and would not have happened without the love, dedication, and support of several very special people.

Firstly, I would like to thank Dr. Angela Lauria, without whom I would not have had the courage to put pen to paper and write this book. No doubt I would have written *a* book, but not this book. She held a mirror to my face when I most needed it and challenged my perceptions about true service.

This is also to Mark Halliday, who told me I would be writing this book six months before I knew it myself.

There are three very special women in my life, whose unwavering love and support means more to me than I can express in words. To Eugenie, to Karolyne, and to Sabine.

My special thanks goes to my mother and step-father, whose generosity, love, and support have completely blown my mind.

None of this would mean anything if I could not share it with my beautiful daughters Mia and Talia, who are the light of my life and whose patience with me went well beyond their years as I wrestled with this book and myself. And of course, to Steve, my long-suffering husband, who must be one of the most patient people on the planet. I love you all!

To the Morgan James Publishing team: Special thanks to David Hancock, CEO & Founder for believing in me and my message. To my Author Relations Manager, Margo Toulouse thanks for making the process seamless and easy. Many more thanks to everyone else, but especially Jim Howard, Bethany Marshall, and Nickcole Watkins.

And lastly, to you, my reader.

I understand the courage it takes to take a long, hard look at life as we find it and change it according to our deepest desires.

About the Author

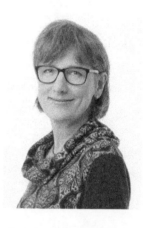

Dr. Maritta Philp, MD, had been working as a doctor for over 20 years before the intensity and stress of modern medical practice inspired her to take a long, hard look at where the road she was on would lead. She realized the final destination for her would be one of burn-out and resentment, causing her to make different choices for her life and career.

Having been interested in psychology, philosophy, and the power of the mind for many years, she gained further qualifications as a hypno-psychotherapist and Rapid Transformational Therapist.

She now works as a successful coach and therapist, helping people to identify and overcome their own obstacles, enabling them to step into a self-directed and empowered life, both personally and professionally.

Maritta is passionate about enabling people to create a life they can be in love with, a life that reflects their most important ideas and values.

She also runs workshops and gives talks on this and related subjects.

She has a no-nonsense and practical approach to life, which is reflected in her work.

Born in Germany, Maritta moved to the UK in 1996 to complete her specialist training. She moved to Scotland soon after, where she still lives with her husband, two beautiful daughters, and her dog Maisie.

Website: www.marittaphilp.com
Email: maritta.philp@gmail.com

Thank You!

Thanks for reading my book. I know you are ready for change, the fact that you have come this far is proof of that.

I know from personal experience how daunting this can be, and I want to do everything in my power to help you in this process.

I have created several tools for you free of charge, all of which you can download from my website at <u>www.marittaphilp.com</u>.

- There is an enlightening questionnaire called "Should I Quit My Practice?" that you can complete. This might give you important insights as to where you are right now.
- There are several worksheets to go with the exercises in the book for you to use.
- In addition to the above, I would be delighted to connect with you through a free strategy session, especially if you want to explore working with me personally.

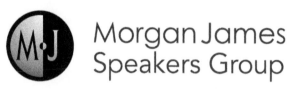

Morgan James
Speakers Group

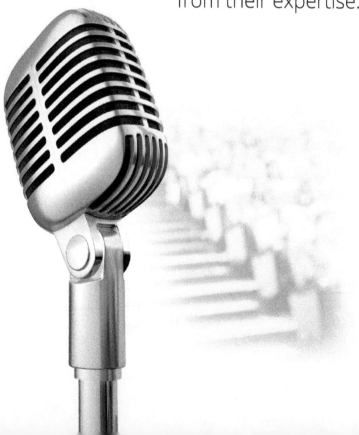

www.TheMorganJamesSpeakersGroup.com

We connect Morgan James published authors with live and online events and audiences who will benefit from their expertise.

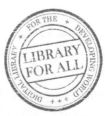

Morgan James makes all of our titles available
through the Library for All Charity Organization.

www.LibraryForAll.org

Printed in the USA
CPSIA information can be obtained
at www.ICGtesting.com
JSHW082351140824
68134JS00020B/2018